Yin Tui Na Techniques
for
Treating Injuries
of
Parkinson's Disease
and
Any Dissociated Injury

Other books by Dr. Janice Hadlock, DAOM

Tracking the Dragon
Recovery from Parkinson's
Medications of Parkinson's Disease or Once Upon a Pill

Yin Tui Na Techniques
for
Treating Injuries
of
Parkinson's Disease
and
Any Dissociated Injury

Dr. Janice Hadlock, DAOM, LAc

Table of contents

Introduction

This book teaches the hands-on therapeutic techniques – the types of Yin Tui Na – that the Parkinson's Recovery Project uses in the treatment of Parkinson's disease.

Tui Na is pronounced "tway nah," as if to rhyme with "Hey! Ma."

"Tui Na" doesn't translate easily into a specific English term. It is often translated, inaccurately, as massage. A more accurate translation would be "any form of hands-on body work." Literally, Tui means push or shove, and Na means hold or take. [1, 2]

Any form of bodywork, whether vigorous or gentle, is called Tui Na. This book teaches *Yin* Tui Na – a subset of Tui Na.

Yin Tui Na might be translated as "those forms of Tui Na that are very subtle, gentle, slow, with movements that might not even be visible to the naked eye." We use a collection of Yin Tui Na techniques when treating people with Parkinson's disease (PD)

What makes a technique "Tui Na" is the application of the practitioner's hands.

The practitioner might be touching the patient's bare skin *or* be working through several layers of the patient's clothing. The practitioner might use bare hands or, if concerned about infectious disease, might wear protective gloves.

Yin Tui Na can be used to treat *any* syndromes resulting from unhealed injury, but this book will focus on its applications for people with Parkinson's. This book is an adjunct to a larger book, *Recovery from Parkinson's*. Originally, the contents of this book were included between the covers of that larger book but, when *Recovery from Parkinson's* grew to be a monster of more than 650 pages, steps had to be taken. [3]

Those steps consisted of moving these instructions for the hands-on, therapeutic treatment that we perform on people with Parkinson's from the larger book into this stand-alone book. Also, a new chapter was written for this book that provides introductory material about Parkinson's disease for people who stumble across this book without having first read the main tome. Also, a chapter that explains the pronunciation and literal meaning of the term Yin Tui Na, and a bit more about the history of this type of medicine, was added at the back of the book.

The techniques in this book were chosen for the treatment of people with Parkinson's because they best help a person bring his mental, emotional and somatic (feeling of

---

[1] The Pinyin Chinese-English Dictionary. Commercial Press. Hong Kong. 1979. p.698

[2] Although the title of the official Chinese government's English translation of the official Tui Na textbook is *Chinese Massage*, most of the techniques of Tui Na, both Yin and Yang types, bear little or no relation to massage, as we understand massage in the west. *Chinese Massage*. Publishing House of Shanghai College of Traditional Chinese Medicine. Shanghai. 1988.

[3] For more detailed information about Parkinson's disease in general, treatment for the mental/emotional components of Parkinson's, and an explanation of recovery symptoms from an old injury from which a person has dissociated – symptoms which can sometimes be unpleasant and even painful – please read *Recovery from Parkinson's*, available for free download at www.pdrecovery.org.

As an aside, *Recovery from Parkinson's* was, for several years, released under the title *Trouble Afoot*, but has been restored to its original title.

sensations in the body) focus to a long-standing, unhealed injury – so that the injury can begin to heal. In the realm of Chinese medicine, these types of techniques fit under the large umbrella term "Yin Tui Na," which itself fits under the vast umbrella term "Tui Na."

Again, the techniques in this book may also prove helpful in the treatment of *any* unhealed injury, whether long-standing or recent, whether presenting in a person with or without Parkinson's disease. The material in this text is the same material I've taught to acupuncture students in the Yin Tui Na class at the local acupuncture college, a class in which students learn Yin Tui Na for *many* situations involving physical injury.

For example, these techniques are used with great success for the setting of broken bones. In fact, Tui Na, historically, was also referred to as "bone medicine." The various techniques of both Yin and Yang types of Tui Na were used over a range of structural (bone and tissue) problems, ranging from the visually obvious, physical (Yang) repositioning of overtly displaced *unbroken* bones to the extremely subtle work (Yin) of supporting broken bones and/or displaced soft tissue so that they reposition *themselves* back into correct alignment.

Parenthetically, some people understandably assume that the term "Chinese bone medicine" refers to the use of petrified bones in medicinal teas. For certain medical conditions, old bones are ground up and boiled in order to deliver calcium and other trace, biologically-bound, minerals for patients deficient in these nutrients. But the classical Chinese term "bone medicine" refers to the certain types of Tui Na, both Yin (subtle) and Yang (overt) that are used for structural realignment work on bones, tendons, ligaments, and fascia.

These techniques can also be helpful for almost any physical injury, whether new and painful or old and painless. Injuries ranging from concussion to badly stubbed toe can usually benefit from treatment with Yin Tui Na.

In my many years as an acupuncturist, I've seen that most patients recover far faster from their injuries or physical pains if some Yin Tui Na precedes the administration of acupuncture. Very often, after the Yin Tui Na work is finished, the pain of the injury is gone *and* the channel Qi has restored itself to its correct pathway – eliminating the need for any acupuncture needles at all.

Yin Tui Na is a valuable medical tool, one that every acupuncturist – and every person – should have in his repertoire.

Whether you are an acupuncturist, a hands-on therapist, or a support person for someone with Parkinson's disease, I hope you will enjoy this book – and maybe someday write your own book about your experiences with Yin Tui Na. In this way, awareness of this ancient medicine can continue to thrive and prosper.

Chapter one

Why use Yin Tui Na for treating Parkinson's disease?

A traumatic injury from which a person has dissociated will not fully heal. Only when the injured person can bring himself to fully acknowledge the injury and its accompanying pain, will the injury be able to heal completely. The most effective treatment for such injuries is often firm, manual support that is non-invasive and non-manipulative: Yin Tui Na

Overview of the techniques we use

The first technique discussed in this book, Forceless, Spontaneous Release, or FSR, instructs in a certain *tempo* of treatment (slow), amount of *pressure* applied with one's hands (firm), and a *lack* of intention that the practitioner brings to the treatment. The physical and emotional support provided by this technique can bring a patient's attention to an injured area so that healing can begin.

FSR can be performed almost anywhere on the body that has unhealed injuries. In people with Parkinson's, the legs, feet, and ankles are areas that nearly always call out for treatment.

This technique does *not* apply particular vectors, directions of movement, to the patient. However, corrective movement in twisted or displaced tissues often occurs, spontaneously, as the patient responds to the firm support. This technique can also be used diagnostically, to detect injuries and holding patterns.

The second technique discussed uses very gentle nudges to suggest directional movements in muscles that have become stuck in a particular holding pattern. The examples of this technique included in this book show applications for the rotational joints of the hips and shoulders, but this technique of gentle nudges can be used in almost any body part that has become locked up. This particular technique does not have a name. It uses the tempo and support principles of FSR, but has intentional movement.

The third technique, craniosacral therapy, is a method for improving and regulating the flow of cerebrospinal fluid via correcting displaced cranial and spinal bones or micro-muscle holding patterns in the joints of these bones. To assist in healthy movement of cerebrospinal fluid, gentle, directional pressures are applied at the various cranial and spinal joint articulations. The vectors for the induced movements at these articulations are highly specific, and are aimed at maximizing the openness of these joints.

This book describes the hand positions and a few of the vector directions most commonly used in craniosacral therapy. However, in treating injuries from which a person has become dissociated, or in people with PD, we combine the very specific hand placements of craniosacral therapy with the FSR tempo, degree of hand pressure, and the *lack* of direction and intention, as opposed to using the usual craniosacral therapy directional forces.

The "minimal," directional nudging used in most styles of craniosacral therapy is, very often, perceived as manipulative and threatening by many people with Parkinson's.

Finally, this book teaches an extremely gentle, or "Yin" technique for releasing psoas muscle spasms – a spasm that is not uncommon in people with Parkinson's disease. Many techniques have been developed for releasing psoas muscle spasms. The particularly Yin method that we use, which people can even do on themselves, gets less emotional resistance from people with Parkinson's than the more traditional but brutal, sometimes even pain-inducing, methods for releasing these spasms.

A brief introduction to Forceless, Spontaneous Release

The Forceless, Spontaneous Release technique is *extremely* "Yin": passive, firm, often motionless, with no "intention" on the part of the practitioner.

The technique consists of this: the vicinity of the patient's unhealed injury is held firmly between the two hands of the therapist, which have been firmly placed on the skin or the clothing on opposite sides of the injured area.

The *two hands don't do anything* except hold, firmly, until such time as the patient's subconscious starts to feel safe enough to pay attention to the area being held, at which point the patient's injured area starts to *move on its own* – often in motions suggesting the (long-delayed) follow-through response to the original injury or motions that suggest relaxation of long-held tension. During these movements, the therapist keeps his firm, supportive hands (usually the palms) pressing on the patient's skin or clothing, while allowing his hands to be carried along by the spontaneous movements being made by the patient.
That's it.

Sounds too simple? Much of this book is spent explaining what is meant in the above paragraph by terms like "firmly," "don't do anything," "move on its own," and all the other terms and questions that arise when doing this extremely non-invasive work on a person who has dissociated from an injury, thus preventing that injury from completely healing.

But first, to understand why the FSR tempo and absence of intention, whether applied to the legs, feet, rotational joints or to the hand positions of craniosacral therapy, is particularly effective for treating people with Parkinson's, one must understand the underlying causes of idiopathic Parkinson's. If you're already familiar with the Chinese channel theory understanding of Parkinson's disease, skip ahead to chapter two. If not, grab a snack and settle in.

The electrical presentation of Parkinson's disease

People with idiopathic Parkinson's disease (PD) and psychogenic parkinsonism (as opposed to drug- or toxin-induced parkinsonism) have a particular electrical pattern running throughout their bodies. This pattern is a *normal* feature of a rarely used neurological mode called "dissociation."[1]

---

[1] Regrettably, the field of psychology also uses the term "dissociation" to describe a completely different phenomenon: the compartmentalization of specific memories, in order to keep them away from normal consciousness. This is *psychological* dissociation. (Continued on next page.)

Dissociation mode usually occurs when a person (or any mammal) experiences a dangerously high level of blood loss, significant puncturing of the skin, loss of limb, or almost any potentially-mortal injury.

In biological dissociation, the "last-gasp attempt at death-prevention" neurological mode, heart rate is *greatly* reduced, breathing rate is *greatly* reduced, blood is pulled away from the skin and shunted deep inside to the spine and brain, blood pressure becomes very low (preventing the further loss of blood), adrenaline and dopamine release is severely inhibited and a surge of endorphins is released. The skin can become cold, and the body may curl up slightly into a fetal position. The person, whether conscious or appearing to be unconscious, may perceive himself from a location that seems to be outside of his own body: hence the name, "dissociation."

(Continued from previous page.) The term "dissociation," or "biological dissociation," as used by animal behaviorists, some biologists, and medical doctors, refers to one of the four autonomic neurological modes: parasympathetic, sympathetic, sleep, and dissociation. Depending on external circumstances and mindset, a person's body chooses the mode, or combination of modes, that is best suited for the activity and mindset of the moment. The neurological mode of the moment determines heart rate, breathing rate, neurotransmitter levels and blood distribution patterns, and other physiological functions for that moment. Parasympathetic mode, the dopamine-driven mode, occurs when a person is awake and feeling good. Sympathetic mode is popularly known as the "fight or flight," or "adrenaline-driven" mode. Most people, during waking hours, are using a mix of parasympathetic and sympathetic modes.

For example, if a person is driving in traffic (a sympathetic mode function primarily regulated by adrenaline) while eating (a parasympathetic mode function regulated by dopamine), he is simultaneously using nerve patterns and neurotransmitters characteristic of *both* parasympathetic mode and sympathetic mode.

The blend of parasympathetic and sympathetic occurs along a continuum: as a person feels more content or more joyful, his body moves closer to the parasympathetic end of the continuum. At this end of the spectrum, his digestion works the best, and his heart rate is fairly low. Dopamine is the dominant neurotransmitter of this mode. As a person becomes more worried or fearful, his body moves closer to the sympathetic end of the spectrum. Blood flows away from the digestive organs and is shunted to the skeletal muscle. Heart rate increases. Adrenaline is the neurotransmitter for this mode.

As one becomes fearful, he instantly moves away from the purely-parasympathetic end of the spectrum and edges closer to the purely-sympathetic. When this happens, adrenaline levels increase and dopamine levels decrease. When he relaxes, he quickly moves back towards the purely-parasympathetic end of the spectrum. Most people, while awake, are almost always somewhere in the *middle* of this spectrum.

As for "sleep" mode, both adrenaline *and* dopamine levels drop very low during this mode, although dreams can trigger the release of mild amounts of these neurotransmitters.

"Dissociation" mode, also sometimes referred to as *biological* dissociation to differentiate it from psychological dissociation, will be discussed at length in this chapter.

For now, consider that the original use of the word "dissociation" had to do with social groups, particularly religious groups. When one left his previous religious group, he was said to have disassociated.

Today, the words dissociated and dis*a*ssociated are used interchangeably, and the most *common* modern usage of "dissociation" refers to psychological dissociation. However, biological dissociation is the type of dissociation referred to in this text, unless otherwise specified.

For a good visual image of dissociation, think of the possum that curls up, looking dead, at the first sign of danger. The possum does not "pretend" to be dead. He cannot help himself. He isn't designed for the "fight or flight" of sympathetic mode: he is uniquely hardwired to slide into dissociation at the first sign of danger.

Another common example of dissociation that many of us have seen occurs when a cat catches a mouse. When the cat's claws perforate the mouse's skin – a significant level of skin perforation can be a trigger for dissociation mode – the mouse becomes rigid, and appears dead: his breathing becomes imperceptible, and his tiny claws curl in in what looks like the rigor mortis of death.

If the cat was hunting for sport, and not hunger, he may bat the rigid mouse around for a few minutes and then, becoming bored, depart in search of livelier prey. About ten minutes later, the mouse will come out of his dissociated state, take a deep breath, shudder from his head all the way down to his tail, (thus resetting his body to his usual blend of parasympathetic and sympathetic modes), and scamper off.

A person, when in *full-blown* dissociated mode, becomes very still, even rigid. The fingers curl in, the skin temperature drops and the body assumes a mild-to-full blown fetal posture. The release of brain dopamine is inhibited. This mode is *usually* of short duration. Either the person dies from the injury, or he soon recovers enough to come out of the dissociated state. If he recovers, he may go through various "shock" related symptoms, such as tremoring, poor temperature regulation, inhibited digestion (including nausea or vomiting), and so on, as his body adjusts back towards the more customary neurological modes: parasympathetic (not fearful), or sympathetic ("fight or flight") or, most likely, a blend of the two.[1]

On a historical note, back in the 1800s, primitive research done on spinal nerves in frogs led biologists to assume that only one neurological mode existed: sympathetic mode. Later, two modes, parasympathetic and sympathetic, were recognized (in western medicine), but it was believed that only one mode could be active at any given time. This very limited, mechanical thinking about neurological modes is reflected in our speech: "Oh, he's in fight-or-flight mode." The idea that only one mode could be active at any given time was still being taught in western medical schools as recently as the 1980s.

Where Asian medicine comes into all this

Each of the neurological modes creates a highly specific electrical pattern throughout the body, including in the detectable electrical flow in the tissues just below the skin. By

---

[1] In Chinese medicine, the existence of four modes (usually translated as "four seasons") was mentioned in the classic text, *Su Wen*, written approximately two thousand years ago. The four "seasons" were described as changes related to 1) "being in tune with the Divine Being" (parasympathetic: physically and mentally relaxed and healthy), 2) "enables us to flee from death" (sympathetic flight or flight), and 3)"stay close to life" (dissociation). The fourth season, sleep, seems to have disappeared from the classic texts over the centuries, because the stanza begins by mentioning "four seasons," and then goes on to list only three.

These quotes from the *Su Wen*, chapter 13-9, are taken from *A Complete Translation of the Yellow Emperor's Classics of Internal Medicine and the Difficult Classic*, Henry C. Lu, PhD, International College of Traditional Chinese Medicine, Vancouver, BC, Canada, 2004.

learning to feel for these patterns, a health practitioner can ascertain just what modes the patient is using at the moment, *and* even discern if various modes are being used, simultaneously, in various, *localized* body parts.

Thousands of years ago, Chinese medicine philosophers were already aware of the electrical pattern differences between parasympathetic, sympathetic, dissociative, and sleep modes. The essence of Chinese medicine is based on an understanding of these electrical patterns, sometimes translated as "the flow of Qi" or "the flow of channel Qi". The maps of the electrical channels that are studied in schools of Chinese medicine even today show the electrical schematics of a healthy, contented, awake person: a person in pure parasympathetic mode.

Details regarding the changes, or divergent patterns, that occur when a person slides into the other neurological modes are detailed in the ancient Chinese classics. These mode-based changes are usually described as "divergences" from the norm, to emphasize that the most correct, healthiest patterns are the "standard," or parasympathetic flow patterns.

People with illness, injury, significant scar tissue, emotional problems, or psychological dissociations that prevent sensory awareness of some body part, will manifest pathological divergent variations in their electrical currents, variations set in motion by the pathology.

By feeling, with our hands, the variations in a patient's currents, we know that, contrary to modern western thought, a person is rarely in only one neurological mode: "only parasympathetic," "only sympathetic," or "only dissociated." We can ascertain, by simply feeling the aberrations in the electrical currents that run just under the skin that, for example, even if *many* of the patient's currents are flowing in the parasympathetic pattern, other body areas *can* be simultaneously manifesting electrical diversions to supply sympathetic mode needs, or presenting aberrant (pathological) patterns in localized areas.

These aberrant patterns may be due to injury or localized infection. They can even be snatches of sympathetic, sleep, or dissociation flow patterns that got "stuck." Such flow patterns might have been needed at some point in time, but if some sections of the flow failed to switch back to parasympathetic when the crisis ended, they might now be causing physiological pathologies.

The basic goal of Asian medicine treatments is usually expressed as "restoring harmony." Harmony, in this usage, means, "getting all the channel Qi to flow in the patterns of parasympathetic mode." This understanding is also expressed, by practitioners of Chinese medicine, as "Go through: no pain, No go through: pain." In this phrasing, "Go through" means: the channel Qi flows in the correct patterns for parasympathetic mode – the patterns we learn in school.[1]

---

[1] Most *modern* acupuncturists, especially most Chinese modern acupuncturists, do not think in terms of channels, even while intoning the classic rubrics such as "Go through: no pain." This is a political situation. Channel theory was denounced and discarded by the communist leaders of China. Because the very idea of channels of energy was mocked by western physicians, the Chinese government banned it. Most people who learn Chinese medicine today learn how to correct aberrations in the channels via acupuncture, but they do not even realize that this is what they are doing: they are locked into vague vocabularies such as "restoring harmony."

The electrical patterns that run just under the surface of the skin are extremely easy to feel by hand. At the acupuncture school where I teach, most students, within a few hours, can start to feel the sensations given off by these currents. Within a few weeks, they are usually able to pick up on subtleties that allow them to distinguish between the currents running just under the skin, deeper currents that run in the muscular fascia, and the deepest currents that run through the fascia that covers the bones. So these currents are *not* arcane or hard to detect.

Most animals are extremely sensitive to these currents: when an animal knows to lick another animal or human "just where the problem is," it's because he's picking up the highly obvious (to him) electrical static that occurs in any place where injury, cellular aberration, or localized infection is causing static-rich aberrations in channel Qi flow. Humans, too, have an innate ability to easily discern these static-discharging problem areas – but our cultural upbringing usually inhibits our ability to detect them.

Dissociation's electrical patterns

The dissociation patterns are *extremely* different from the usual electrical patterns that flow under the skin, and are very easy to feel. In many cases, when a person is dissociated, some of the largest currents even flow *backwards*. But even if a person doesn't know which direction the currents are supposed to flow, and therefore doesn't know if the current is flowing backwards or not, it's still easy to tell if the currents of a fellow human are running in the dissociation pattern: the dissociation patterns just feel *wrong*; when you detect them in another person, they might even, in severe cases, make your skin crawl or make your hairs stand on end.

During dissociation, the flow of the electrical current on the outer (lateral) side of the leg (a section of the electrical path known as the Stomach Channel) becomes altered in such a way that it may feel as if the flow is *reversed*, or possibly going *back and forth*, or even, in severe cases, completely *gone*. Even if one doesn't know which direction the energy is supposed to flow, the backwards-flowing or back-and-forth energy gives off a strange, unhealthy, static-rich electromagnetic field. If the energy is missing altogether, it can feel positively creepy to the person assessing the channel Qi; it can seem as if the person's leg is somehow dead.

*

Here's the gist: *The electrical flow patterns of dissociation are a perfect match for the electrical flow patterns that can be easily detected in people with Parkinson's disease.*[1]

*

The medicine has become, to a great extent, formulaic: for problem "X", use this treatment "X". The changes that occur in response to the treatments, changes that restore health by correcting the flow of channel Qi, are often not recognized by modern acupuncturists as having *anything* to do with channel Qi.

[1] For instructions on learning how to feel the flow of Channel Qi, please read the material on this subject – downloadable for free – at www.pdrecovery.org. The free material is excerpted from an acupuncture class text, *Tracking the Dragon*.

What causes the electrical patterns of Parkinson's disease – patterns that resemble the patterns of dissociation?

Well, that depends on the individual. Several factors other than mortal injury and impending death can cause electrical patterns similar to those of dissociation.

1) A foot and/or ankle injury that blocks the terminus of the Stomach channel (on the top center of the foot) can cause backwards-flowing energy in the Stomach channel (which, in health, flows *down* the lateral side of the leg, *from* the hip *towards* the toes). This backwards flow can, over time, cause disruptions in other channels. When the channel aberrations get to the point where they disrupt the channels that run over the head, thus creating patterns that very nearly *mimic the electrical pattern of biological dissociation*, they will automatically trigger the inhibition of dopamine release and the other changes characteristic of biological dissociation.

(The detailed electrical schematics of this foot injury-based dopamine inhibition and an explanation of how the electrical disarray snowballs over time is provided in *Recovery from Parkinson's.*[1])

2) A particular psychological attitude – the one invoked by people with powerful self-control in order to induce numbness to one's own physical or emotional pain, either in one specific part of the body, or body-wide, can set in motion an alteration in the electrical flow in the connective tissue around the heart (the pericardium) and altered signals in some of the neurons in the heart itself.

This mentally induced inhibition of the sensory-awareness function of the pericardium/heart will set in motion the dissociation-style flow of Channel Qi in the area of the heart and pericardium. This mental inhibition, if sustained, will eventually cause more and more of the body's channels to adopt the same electrical flow patterns that are seen during dissociation – a pattern that causes inhibition of dopamine release, stiffness, backwards flow of channel Qi in the legs, and other changes characteristic of Parkinson's disease.

3) Both: In people with idiopathic Parkinson's, the dissociation-like electrical flow might have been set in motion by a foot/ankle injury that causes a blockage at or near the terminus of the Stomach channel, *or* by becoming mentally impervious to one's own pain via altering the electrical flow in the pericardium/heart, or, *most often*, by both.

Note: for ease of writing and reading, from now on I will simply say "dissociation from the heart," rather than "dissociation from the pericardium/heart."

In our research, working with hundreds of people with Parkinson's disease, we have seen that about five percent of our patients have an unhealed foot injury, an injury from which they have *psychologically* dissociated so that it cannot heal *and* no mentally induced dissociation *other* than dissociation from the foot injury (no heart dissociation).

---

[1] *Recovery from Parkinson's* by Janice Hadlock is available for free download at www.pdrecovery.org.

Oppositely, two percent of our patients have no unhealed foot injury or other significant injury, but do recall making a conscious decision to become impervious to physical or emotional pain.

The rest of our patients have both situations: they have a foot injury from which they have psychologically dissociated, so that the injury has never healed, and they also have availed themselves of the mentally-induced trick of turning off their ability to feel the heart response to their own physical or emotional pain. They may be highly sensitive to the pain of *others*, or they might not be. Perception of and compassion for pain in *others* has nothing to do with dopamine inhibition. The perception that is inhibited in people with Parkinson's is the awareness of the physiological signals that tell of pain originating in their *own* bodies.[1]

In some of these patients, the heart numbing is extreme: they may not have *any* idea what is meant by the phrase "My heart expanded with joy." They may have no memory of ever experiencing the feeling of expansion in the chest that occurs when one relaxes, hears beautiful music, or "warms" to a charming scene.

In other patients, the heart numbing comes and goes: if you tell them a joke, or if they feel, momentarily, utterly safe, they cease to dissociate from the heart. They relax. The electrical flow in their legs temporarily flows in a normal pattern. Their Parkinson's symptoms may temporarily disappear. But as soon as they remember to be wary or self-conscious, the electrical flow in their legs immediately resumes the dissociation patterns. The flow stops or reverses, mimicking the patterns seen in mortal-injury dissociation and in Parkinson's disease.

The relationship between dissociation and dopamine

The electrical patterns set in motion by a long-term unhealed foot injury *or* by heart numbness can, correctly, cause the inhibition of dopamine release. It is *correct* and *normal* for dopamine release to be inhibited when one is in a dissociated condition.

When, as in most cases of PD, dopamine release is minimized or highly inhibited over *decades*, the cells in the area in the brain that create dopamine can slowly, over those decades, long prior to the appearance of PD symptoms, revert back to somewhat "neutral" cells. These brain cells are not dead, but they are no longer functioning as dopamine-producing cells. This is the status of the substantia nigra cells in people with idiopathic Parkinson's disease.[2]

---

[1] People with Parkinson's *can* feel a particular type of pain – the pain that comes from structural rigidity. This pain comes from muscles that have become over-tight. These pains seem to be processed differently from the pains of unhealed injury. Even if a person with Parkinson's always had a "high tolerance" for pain, he will not have a high tolerance for *this* type of pain. I suspect that this type of excess muscle tension pain is handled by a different part of the brain from injury-based pain, or is in some other way different from the pain of injury. Possibly, these pains are processed, in the brain, in a manner similar to arthritis pain, which is processed *not* in the pain area of the brain but, oddly enough, in the fear area of the brain.

Or possibly, as the dissociation becomes chronic and overarching, the accompanying release of endorphins ebbs, making the person susceptible to pain. I just don't know.

[2] "In Parkinson's disease...although dopamine is depleted, the cells in the striatum are *preserved*. This is unlike the PD-like disorders [drug- and toxin- induced parkinsonism] where, in the striatum, the dopamine content is decreased and the cells are *lost*." [Italics mine.] Dr. A. Lieberman, MD, National Medical Director, National Parkinson's Foundation, Inc.; *Parkinson's Report*, Fall 2000, p. 10.

The body is very efficient. If there is no call for dopamine, the dopamine-producing cells eventually become dormant, and then revert back to what is known as "undifferentiated cells" (early embryo-type cells). They cease to be dark-colored ("nigra") cells.

As an aside, during the many years prior to the appearance of Parkinson's disease symptoms, while the dopamine release is inhibited and dopamine cells are reverting to "neutral" cells, people with latent (not yet visible) Parkinson's usually use *adrenaline*, not dopamine, for thought and motor function.

Usually, a person's Parkinson's symptoms *appear*, his symptoms become visible, when his ability to summon up adrenaline for all the mundane chores of daily living begins to taper off.

Those of our patients who have recovered from Parkinson's, who start moving via dopamine instead of adrenaline, are usually shocked at how wonderful and utterly different it feels to move using dopamine instead of adrenaline. They often say that they don't remember *ever* having moved in such an effortless manner. They've always moved in a more "conscious" way: using adrenaline – which requires a different type of mental instruction than dopamine motor function.

For example, in getting up off a sofa, a person using *adrenaline* will think to himself, "Get off the sofa." He may even mentally think through the steps involved: "Push down with your hands, extend the torso forward, push the butt up and straighten the spine." These thoughts will be lightening fast instructions, and practically automatic. He will *think* of the processes involved. The person will not start by imagining what it *feels* like to stand up.

But when a person who is using primarily *dopamine* thinks, "I want to stand up," his mind, lightening fast, *imagines* what that will *feel* like: the *sensations* of the muscles, the *sensations* of changing his position. He does *not* issue mental instructions. The next thing he knows, he is standing. This process is performed in the motor imagining area of the brain – an area that is off-limits during dissociation, and which also happens to be off-limits in people with Parkinson's disease.[1]

Hence, the need to use adrenaline in the years of latent (pre-) Parkinson's.

Some examples of dissociation-related behaviors from basic injury

If these concepts are very new to the reader, he might be saying to himself that injuries can't possibly cause an alteration in brain neurotransmitter release. The following example might be helpful.

A *short-term* electrical aberration that is very similar to that of dissociation can *correctly* occur, immediately, in response to a significant leg or foot injury, such as a broken or grossly displaced bone in the leg. A person who has *just* broken his leg may experience some degree of dissociation-like symptoms such as rigidity, certainly a decreased desire to move, tightening of, and even numbness in, the toes and fingers, the body pulling into a mild fetal position, a feeling of withdrawal from sensory input, decreased appetite, poor temperature regulation (cold or clammy skin or hot flashes) poor speech production, and so on. These specific changes occur because of the immediate alterations in his body's electrical circuitry, which, in turn, cause his brain's dopamine release to be greatly inhibited.

---

[1] Research using fSPECT scans (real-time imaging of brain activity) has proven that the motor imagining area in people with fairly one-sided Parkinson's symptoms is inactive for the side of the body with symptoms. This subject is discussed and referenced in *Recovery from Parkinson's*.

Then again, if he *needs* to move to get himself to safety, he will be able to do so easily, even painlessly, by using adrenaline, *even if his leg is broken*. But once he finds himself in a safe place and the adrenaline turns off, the dissociated mode will be the dominant mode – due to the severe foot/leg injury – and this mode's lack of adrenaline and dopamine, together with the specific electrical-flow patterns of dissociation mode, will cause him to assume a rigid posture, somewhat hunched forward, low blood pressure, and other symptoms typical of dissociation – and of Parkinson's.

A few hours after the leg was broken, when the patient is in a safe place and no longer needing to "run from the lion" or "perform" for the doctor (a performance powered by adrenaline), the patient might notice the onset of some of the symptoms mentioned previously: he may become somewhat withdrawn, shivering, curled up, not hungry, his skin may be cool to the touch, and his breathing and heart rate might be diminished – like the mouse whose skin was perforated by the claws of a cat. If so, he may also feel somewhat numb to the pain. Depending on his symptoms, we might even say he is in "shock."

The currents in the patient's leg will be physically disrupted at the point of the leg break. The leg current, unable to flow past the break, will either shunt into a nearby, unaffected current, or it will run backwards.

If it runs backwards, his body probably will manifest some symptoms of dissociation, including dopamine inhibition, until the injury heals to the point where electrical current can once again flow correctly: flowing past, or around, the injury, and following the parasympathetic (healthy) route.

– As an aside, in 1817, James Parkinson noted in his monograph, *An Essay on the Shaking Palsy* [Parkinson's disease], that people with the shaking palsy are able to move *perfectly normally* during a true emergency, and their shaking palsy symptoms only return when the emergency ends.

This observation has been repeatedly confirmed in modern times: during a true emergency, the tremors and rigidity of Parkinson's disease will temporarily cease, as the body becomes flooded with adrenaline. Just as a person with a broken leg can run for miles on that broken leg if he is being chased by a lion, a person with advanced Parkinson's can flee from a burning house – moving perfectly normally. But as soon as he is out of the emergency situation, the Parkinson's rigidity will return. Even if the body's electrical circuits are *usually* moving in the dissociation pattern, which is the case in Parkinson's, the release of adrenaline can over-ride the rigidity that comes from dissociation-based dopamine inhibition *IF* the dopamine inhibition was mentally induced – which it is, in most cases of idiopathic Parkinson's. Again, so long as the dissociation is psychologically induced, an adrenaline surge can always over-ride the dissociation: hence, people with PD can mask their absence of dopamine release by maintaining mental or physical intensity in their life-style.

Oppositely, in cases of biological dissociation caused by on-going, near-death trauma such as *severe* loss of blood or *severe* penetration of the skin, adrenaline-based behaviors might *not* be available: the *dangerously* injured person may not be able to override the dissociation with adrenaline. He may even slide into loss of consciousness.

Getting back to our example of a person with a broken leg, his dissociation-like symptoms will cease as soon as he begins to heal – sometimes, even as soon as he *decides* that he is in a safe place and is *going* to start healing.

Very little healing occurs while a person is in dissociated mode. Healing primarily occurs when a person feels safe – when he is in parasympathetic mode or sleep mode. Once the injured person is able to feel that he's going to be safe after all, or that help is on the way, his thoughts move him in a parasympathetic direction and the symptoms of dissociation ease off. Before sliding completely out of dissociation, and into the parasympathetic/sympathetic continuum, he may go into shock, for a while. Shock is a condition in which one hovers between dissociation and the parasympathetic/sympathetic modes.

But eventually, when he feels safe, inside and out, he will take a deep breath and experience a shudder that goes from the back of his head down to the bottom of his spine. This shudder helps turn the vagus nerve (the dominant nerve of parasympathetic mode) back on and resets the sympathetic mode-based spinal nerves. The person thus turns off the dissociated mode and any related adrenaline-based override, and reverts back to "normal": a blend of parasympathetic and sympathetic modes. The injury can begin to heal.

For another example of a person using his mind to switch neurological modes, consider a swimmer who has gotten chilled while swimming in very cold water. When he gets out of the mountain lake or cold ocean, he finds himself shivering. Still shivering, he makes his way over to his towel. Maybe he sits in the sun. At some point, he will entertain the thought, "I'm OK now" or "I'm safe now." At this point, he will think to himself, "I don't need to be shivering any more."

At that moment, in response to that conscious decision, he will *automatically* take a deep breath, a shudder will pass down his spine, and he will instantly stop shivering. If the chilling was severe, he may find himself doing the "deep breath and shudder" two or three times.

When I describe the above "getting out of cold-water" scenario to my patients with Parkinson's, most of them have no idea what I'm talking about when I describe the "deep breath and shudder." Their spouses, sitting next to them, nod their heads and say, "Oh yes, I know what you mean!"

People with Parkinson's, for the most part, do not know how, or you might say *no longer* know how, to mentally turn off the previously inserted mental conviction that they are at risk – a conviction that, with their powerful minds, directs them to remain dissociated. For various reasons, people with Parkinson's cannot bring themselves to say to themselves, in a convincing manner, "I'm safe now." They usually do not remember any experience of having the deep breath and shudder experience. They do not recall ever having been, firstly, stressed and shaky, and then secondly consciously deciding that they are "OK after all," thus allowing their physiology to revert back to predominantly parasympathetic.

Linking Parkinson's and the electrical pattern of dissociation

Again, what we see in people with Parkinson's is electrical schematics very similar to the electrical patterns that occur naturally during dissociation. However, naturally occurring dissociation patterns are usually very short-term. In Parkinson's disease, they have become chronic.

Our research, over more than a decade, has found that 98% of our patients with idiopathic Parkinson's have an *unhealed* foot/ankle/leg injury. Often, the patient has no recall of any injury, even if the ankle/foot bones are severely displaced, or even showing signs of repairative surgery. The injuries are usually *found* by using FSR, a supportive holding technique that can be *diagnostic*, as well as therapeutic.

In these cases, bones might *still* be severely displaced or broken (the injuries can sometimes be visible in x-rays), even if the injuries occurred decades earlier. Many of the unhealed injuries we've worked on were received in childhood.

Very typically, at the time of injury, the patient was more concerned about some other, more life-threatening situation, and so the injury was ignored. The "life-threatening situation" of the childhood-era injury might have been nothing more than dread fear of mocking friends, or terror that the parents might find out about the injury. Also, many people with Parkinson's were taught, as children, that they should never cry or show vulnerability.

For whatever reason, these people got hurt and decided it was better to not acknowledge the injury: they mentally dissociated from the injury (psychological dissociation). After this, they were able to use adrenaline to enable themselves to move normally even though injured.

Note: this is an aspect of *psychological* dissociation. You will see how this *psychological* dissociation prevents the *healing* of injury. The electrical static that surrounds an unhealed foot/ankle injury sets in motion alterations in the leg's electrical currents – alterations that resemble those of *biological* dissociation.

Essentially, these people told their brain that the injury hadn't happened, or to ignore it. When a person does this, his obedient brain is not able to initiate significant healing processes in the injured area until such time as the psychological dissociation instruction is rescinded. In most of our patients, the actual injury itself seems to have spent decades in a state of suspended animation.

When, *during the application of FSR*, the patient's awareness is finally brought to bear on the injury, together with the support-induced thought, "I'm safe now," the injury might only then manifest its first swelling, bruising, and pain – normal features of the injury that never occurred at the time of the trauma. These features had been held in check by the dissociation.

Until the mental instruction of "deny the pain" is rescinded, the brain maintains a localized zone of *psychological* dissociation. Superficially, it may appear that healing has occurred: the skin, if broken, might quickly have healed over. However, the normal patterns of full healing may not have occurred.

As an aside, the curious reader might find the above proposition extremely far-fetched. However, nearly all of the people with Parkinson's that we have seen have told us that, upon reading the full details about this psychological process and the associated biological changes, they've understood *exactly* what we're describing. They insist that it perfectly describes the way they've felt in their mind and body even during the decades before the Parkinson's symptoms slowly showed up. Many have even said (I paraphrase), "I never thought that anyone could ever understand the strange way I've always felt inside. I always knew I responded to certain physical and/or emotional things differently than other people. It's wonderful to know that there's an explanation for it." And "I'm not alone, after all!"

14

For that matter, we've observed that most of our patients with Parkinson's tend to be highly analytical and highly skeptical of "unproven" science. Even so, most of our PD patients (and their spouses and close friends) have been in absolute agreement with our hypotheses because they see the "unique" characteristics of themselves or, respectively, their loved one with PD, in our detailed descriptions of what it feels like *inside* to have Parkinson's and also what the thoughts of a person with Parkinson's are often like.

We've noticed that people who do not have PD or who do not have a close personal experience of a person with Parkinson's have a harder time accepting that anyone could attain this type of dissociation. They are reluctant to accept this understanding of Parkinson's, an understanding very foreign to the western medical tradition. But when the patients themselves say, with fervor and relief, "It's like you were writing about *me*! For the first time, I felt like someone else knows what I'm like!" it only adds to our confidence in our hypotheses. And having people recover adds to our confidence, as well.

Getting back to the point, the psychological dissociation from the location of the injury creates a problem: an *unhealed* injury in the foot or ankle area can, over time, gradually build up a body-wide electrical pattern that matches the electrical patterns of *biological* dissociation: body-wide patterns that are *supposed* to cause inhibition of dopamine release, and all the other symptoms of Parkinson's disease.

Likewise, generalized, body-wide *psychological* dissociation from the ability to feel one's somatic pain also causes electrical flow that matches the electrical patterns of *biological* dissociation: patterns that are *supposed* to cause inhibition of dopamine release, and all the other symptoms of Parkinson's disease.

In other words, there is some degree of psychological dissociation in people with Parkinson's, either from somatic feeling, in general, or from a specific injury, or both. This dissociation, and the subsequent inability of the injury to heal, causes electrical conditions that mimic the dissociative neurological mode. The electrical patterns of this mode, in turn, trigger the inhibition of dopamine and the subsequent appearance of symptoms that match those of Parkinson's disease.

Not helped by talk therapy

In our research, we've found that this psychologically induced dissociation from the heart, which is to say, dissociation from the ability to *feel* somatic experiences, *cannot* be turned off by mental exercises such as talk therapy or a labored attempt at a mental shift. What does help is an absolute, abrupt shift in attitude: "I'm OK after all" or "I'm perfectly safe, even though I'm *not* in control of anything in my life." No external therapy can force the patient to change his determination to indulge in this mindset.

But the psychological dissociation from the specific *injury*, as opposed to dissociation from the heart, *can* sometimes be terminated via manual treatment. The injury dissociation which can be at the root of the biological dissociation pattern, *can* often be successfully addressed by the very supportive, non-invasive, comfort-giving work of various forms of Yin Tui Na, techniques which encourage the patient to *dare to feel* the injury that he has, for so long, feared to feel.

To treat a case of Parkinson's disease that has been triggered by a foot or ankle injury, the patient's attention must be brought to bear on his still-unhealed injury so that his brain can realize that unfinished business is present *and* that it's safe to now address that injury – even *feel* the injury.

Treating the forms of Parkinson's disease that *also* feature dissociation from the heart usually requires other, self-directed mental change, as well, but this book is focused on the injury portion that can lead to Parkinson's.

Then again, some people with Parkinson's – even those who also have dissociation from the heart – fully recover in response to having their injury treated. It seems as if, in these cases, their heart dissociation was connected to the foot injury. Or maybe, when they decide to *stop* dissociating from one problem, they are able to *stop* other dissociations, as well. At any rate, we've seen people go through physiological as well as psychological changes, and fully recover from Parkinson's, merely by having their injuries treated.

Then again, we've also seen many people who experience only partial recovery after their injuries heal. The injuries heal and their electrical patterns flow in parasympathetic mode – so long as they are feeling completely safe. But at any sign of anxiety or fear, they revert to their fear-based habit of heart dissociation.

In these cases, people might have no symptoms of Parkinson's so long as they are feeling relaxed or at ease, but as soon as any sort of threat arises – such as a trip to the dentist – they lapse back into parkinsonism until the threat is over. These people need to learn how to deal with fear without resorting to dissociating from their "heart." That subject is addressed in the book *Recovery from Parkinson's.*

This book addresses the treatment of unhealed injury.

Bringing the patient's attention to the unhealed injury

We've learned that, as therapists, if we impose any therapy that is deemed even slightly invasive onto the injured/dissociated area, it is usually perceived as threatening. In response to the "threat" of therapy, the patient will automatically increase the level of dissociation in the injured area. So how gentle must a therapy be to prevent it from being "invasive"?

We've learned that, for some people with Parkinson's, even *looking* at their injured area can be a bit too invasive, at first. Touching it is out of the question, at first, for some patients. We might have to work up to supporting the foot injury by firmly holding and supporting the knee or calf for some number of sessions, before slowly easing down towards the foot.

"No, you can't look at my foot"

A middle-aged woman with Parkinson's and her husband drove all the way up from Los Angeles to Santa Cruz, to have me work on her foot. She had read all the material available on our website, and knew that I was going to have to touch her foot. She nervously waited for her turn. After asking all the usual intake questions, I asked her to remove her shoe. She paused a long time, then said, "No. I don't even allow my husband to look at my feet. I can't let you look at my feet."

She burst into tears, apologized for taking up my time, and left. I never saw her again.

Then again, some people with Parkinson's *love* having their poor, neglected foot or leg injuries held and supported, after so many years of ignoring them.

Most people with Parkinson's are somewhere in the middle: they are mildly apprehensive, at first, and eventually grow to enjoy the sensations of having their injured areas held.

Happily, we've seen that, *if* the patient's consciousness *can* be brought to acknowledge the injury, in a manner that is utterly non-threatening, the mind *will* turn off the dissociation – at least in that area – and work with the body to start the healing process. This healing initiation may bring forth swelling, internal bleeding, pain, limping, and all the usual events that should have followed the injury, and which precede the eventual healing of an injury – events that had been put on hold indefinitely – and those events are a good thing.

Have all people with Parkinson's disease dissociated from their injuries to the same extent?

No. Some of our patients *recall* a foot or ankle injury. It might even have been the most painful thing they've ever experienced.

For many others, their injuries – even broken bones still visible in an x-ray – never hurt at all, and do not begin to hurt until they are treated with FSR.

For some of our patients, even in the cases of broken bones, severely displaced bones and torn ligaments and tendons, *at the time of injury* there had been no pain, no swelling, no bruising, or any other physical indication that an injury had occurred.

Many patients have had no recall of *any* injury until, after being diagnosed with Parkinson's, they've had their feet treated with FSR – and as the injury started hurting, preparatory to healing, memories of the injuries came forth.

Many patients have been so surprised at the sudden "appearance" of an injury that they have contacted a family member to inquire about what might have caused it. Often, the family member recalls the patient having had a stunning traumatic injury at that location. The injury, curiously, never seemed to hurt or cause immobility at the time.

The degree of mental dissociation from the injury can be mild, or it can be extremely severe. For example, some *do* recall the injury, but insist that it was "no big deal." This would suggest a mild level of dissociation.

Other patients, when asked, "How or when did you get this huge scar on the top of your foot?" reply, "What scar? Oh! I've never *seen* that before...I have no idea how it got there..." This inability to even see an obvious scar suggests a somewhat higher level of dissociation.

Some patients with scars bordered by *suture* scars, indicating that the area was sewn up by a doctor, have no idea how the scars got there, and have never seen the suture marks or scars on the top of their own feet.

Whether the Parkinson's patient recalls the injury fully, somewhat, or doesn't recall it at all, doesn't matter. In order for it to heal, he needs to bring his full attention to the injury, including his ability to experience the *sensations* of the injury.

During sleep, emergencies, and dissociation, we do not feel the full complement of internal, ongoing sensory (somatic) experiences. When we are primarily in sympathetic mode, we only perceive those sensations that are necessary for safety: *all* sensations, including smell, taste, sound, sight, and tactile feeling, are assessed in terms of personal safety, rather than richness of experience, when a person's *sympathetic* mode functions are dominant.

Only when a person is *predominantly* in parasympathetic mode can he feel to the fullest all the sensations of his body.

To help bring a patient's *full* attention to his injuries, from the viewpoint of *parasympathetic* mode, we use an *extremely* non-invasive type of supportive holding: FSR. The Yin types of Tui Na use extremely gentle manipulation. With basic FSR, there is no manipulation or movement whatsoever.

Basic Questions

How long is a treatment session? How many treatments does a person need to recover from Parkinson's?

The injury-holding sessions in our clinic typically last about an hour. At our clinic, we might see local patients once a week. Patients who are getting treated by friends or family might get treated every day, or a few times a week. Sometimes, when the dissociation starts to ease off and/or the healing starts, a person might want more treatments – or he might only want to be treated once every two weeks or so.

Questions as to the number of sessions required, and whether the patient will need treatments for several weeks or several years, bring up the subject of variability.

What factors play a part in this variability?

The *time frame* that the patient used when he created his dissociation-inducing attitude can be significant.

For example, if the patient, at the time of injury, told himself "I can't deal with this injury *now*, I'll deal with it *later*, " then the patient has mentally set himself up to deal with the pain at a later time. This is good.

The supportive holding of FSR can suggest to the brain, "I'm safe now. Now's the time to finally get around to dealing with this." In other words, in this type of case, the brain has put the problem on hold, but hasn't denied its existence. It might not take too many sessions for this person to start healing.

If the patient, at the time of injury, told himself, "This isn't happening. There is no injury," it will take a lot longer for the supportive holding to trigger recognition and healing in the brain. The lie: "This never happened" may need to be addressed and retracted. Therapy might take a lot longer than if the patient had merely told himself, "Not now." The ego-based part of the brain doesn't like to make retractions. The brain cannot say "I'm safe *now*" if the brain is sticking like glue to the self-deceit, "Nothing bad ever happened."

If the patient, at the time of injury, told himself, "*I* am a person who does not acknowledge pain. *I* do not feel pain," then the patient is going to have his work cut out for himself.

He must correct the thought that he does not feel pain. The truth is, his body *has* recorded and remembered every incidence of pain that he has experienced – but he's compartmentalized those pains into a part of his brain that is inaccessible to normal awareness. Because of this *psychologically-induced* dissociation from his ability to experience somatic pain, he has not had a chance to respond to and heal from the pain.

Meanwhile, his so-called inability to feel pain may have become, over the years, hardened into a conviction that has become intertwined with the patient's self-identity.

When a person successfully tells himself that he doesn't feel pain, period, a particular physiological event occurs: the signals that normally go to the brain from the pericardium and heart tissues become inhibited.

This self-numbing mechanism is difficult to initiate. Typically, a person must have very high levels of mental focus, thought control, and drive, in order to successfully turn off his awareness of his own physical and emotional pain for the long term. It is hard to do. Most people cannot do it.

It's a *good* thing that the conviction of "I do not feel pain" is hard to instill in oneself, because the "I do not feel pain" posture can set in motion the exact same electrical patterns as mortal injury-type dissociation. In fact, the mental attitude of being numb to pain is *closely related* to mortal-injury (*biological-type*) dissociation:

When a person has a life-threatening trauma and his autonomic nervous system slides into the mode of biological dissociation, *he feels no physical or emotional pain.*

You may have heard the old adage, "mortal injuries don't hurt." It's true. Dissociation due to extreme trauma *inhibits* the electrical transmissions from the "central receiving station" of the heart and pericardial tissues over to the brain's conscious awareness station.

In a healthy person, these heart-to-brain transmissions tell the brain *how* to interpret somatic (within the body) feelings of pain and pleasure.

When, due to dire, life-threatening physical or emotional trauma, dissociation kicks in, the pericardium and heart's communication with the brain ceases. Simultaneously, endorphins are released, preventing the transmission of pain signals to the brain via the spinal cord route. Thus, *perception* of pain is halted via two mechanisms: alteration of the radio-like signals from the heart to the brain and the endorphin-induced inhibition of conduction in spinal-nerve impulses.

In the same way, even in the absence of *physical* trauma, *electing* to turn off these heart signals and spinal signals sets in motion the mortal-injury type of alterations in the electrical flows to the brain. The brain then behaves as if dissociated: dopamine release is inhibited, along with many other symptoms of dissociation.

Over decades, this mind-induced pattern can snowball until the "feel no pain" electrical pattern is creating full-blown dissociation – rigidity, inhibition of dopamine release, diminished sensory function, and all the other symptoms of Parkinson's disease. While these symptoms can be overridden by reliance on adrenaline, the symptoms will begin to appear when the adrenaline response, with age, begins to diminish in vigor, or when the person becomes less able to conjure up a constant sense of false emergency.

In other words, biological dissociation from mortal or near-mortal injury creates a condition in which a person feels no pain. Conversely, by telling oneself that he feels no pain, one triggers electrical patterns that are similar to those of near-mortal injury dissociation.[1]

---

[1] You can say that activity between these two systems, the pericardial/heart and the dissociation systems, are reciprocal. In animals, many such reciprocal systems exist. For example, a physical condition can cause a corresponding mental shift. Oppositely, a mental shift can create a matching physical condition. These reciprocities are baffling to practitioners of western medicine, who keep looking for chemical messengers. Western medicine has no system to account for the *mutual* influences of brain and body. In Chinese medicine, we recognize that the electrical flows of channel Qi, flows that are influenced by both physical structures *and* the electromagnetic waves generated by *thoughts*, are responsible for creating many of these reciprocities.

Now, for the average person, just telling himself that he feels no pain is not going to actually prevent him from feeling pain over the long-term. Most people do not have the mental power, or the desire, to actually put into effect a long-term, sustained numbing of somatic awareness.

However, most people with Parkinson's are extremely intelligent and highly focused, with enormous self-control. These qualities may be genetic, they may come from lifetimes of practicing self-discipline – that is not germane to this discussion.

But in our limited experience, nearly all our patients with PD have a ferocious capability for mental focus, determination, self-discipline, and a circumspect way of viewing themselves and their role in life that is extremely different from the average person. In fact, it was their unexpected, peculiar uniformity of *mental* qualities that finally helped us understand fully the processes that were going on in Parkinson's disease.

Getting back to the point, when people with Parkinson's use their highly advanced mental skills to dissociate from pain for the long-term, they are doing themselves a disservice: they are very likely setting in motion the steps that lead to Parkinson's disease. And it can be extremely difficult to retract the long-forgotten command to "be a person who feels no pain."

Does the duration of treatments vary based on what *caused* the Parkinson's?
Good question.

This next section describes the *treatment* ramifications of the three methods of inducing Parkinson's disease. As you will recall, these three PD-inducing methods are:

1) a heart-based posture of dissociation from one's own physical and/or emotional pain: the "feel no pain" attitude

2) a foot injury *plus* a heart-based posture of dissociation: injury *plus* attitude.

3) only a foot injury

The duration of treatment can depend, to some degree, on which of the above three factors the PD patient has, as well as the time-frame specific mental instructions issued when first installing the feel-no-pain attitude, if any. The following discusses the treatment duration related to these three factors.

1) A feel-no-pain attitude
As noted, the pericardial, or *body-wide*, self-numbing method of inducing an electrical system similar to that of dissociation can create Parkinson's disease, *even in the absence of foot or other injury*. Two percent of our hundreds of patients with idiopathic Parkinson's have *not* had foot/ankle injuries, or even significant neck or back or other injuries…but they have admitted to making a *conscious* decision, in childhood, to inhibit their ability to feel, in order to be impervious to physical and emotional pain. In our limited experience, the patients have always done this in response to the death of a parent or very close relatives.

In these cases, where an attitudinal stance is inhibiting the signals from the heart, thus triggering the same type of electrical flows that ordinarily only occur during mortal-wound type dissociation, this mental attitude *must* be retracted before the person can recover from Parkinson's disease.

Retraction of this attitude can take place in a matter of minutes. But summoning up the courage to do it may take years, or lifetimes. Typically, a person who, in childhood, has learned to numb himself to physical and emotional pain has never learned the methods by which an adult processes pain. He is, therefore, terrified of experiencing it. This terror must be willingly overcome, and only the patient himself can bring about this change.

Time frame: extremely variable.

2) An unhealed foot injury *and* a feel-no-pain attitude

A majority of the PD patients that we have worked with 1) have practiced some level of dissociation from the heart and 2) have an unhealed foot/ankle injury.

This section will be a bit lengthy, because this is the most common presentation *and* because most people in this situation keenly want to believe that the foot injury portion is the more significant part of the problem.

In cases where the heart dissociation came first, the presence of an unhealed foot injury just makes sense. Nearly everyone hurts his feet at some time or other: he twists an ankle, kicks an immoveable object, drops something heavy onto the foot, and so on.

If a person has already *developed an emotional stance of being impervious to sensations of his own physical or emotional pain, he will be able to effortlessly dissociate from the foot injury – so that the injury doesn't hurt…and it doesn't heal.*

Thus, he has *two* processes going on in his body that will gradually lead to an electrical system that resembles that of dissociation. First, the heart dissociation will cause an electrical flow that mimics that of mild dissociation. Second, the injury, which he didn't acknowledge because he was already accustomed to dissociating from painful events, will eventually set in motion a steadily increasing backwards electrical flow that also mimics the flow of dissociation.

If you're looking for "original cause," the original cause *might* well be the attitude – if the attitude preceded the foot injury. After all, the attitude, in and of itself, can cause Parkinson's.

Many people with Parkinson's have told us that they've always had a "high threshold for pain," so that, when they injured their foot, "it was no big deal." Such a high threshold for pain would suggest that, even *prior* to the significant foot injury, the feel-no-pain attitude was highly developed.

Oppositely, we've had patients who've instituted dissociation from the heart *because* of or *simultaneous* with the foot injury. An example of this is our patient who had dropped an eighty-pound ammunition box on his foot during a war-time attack in the WWII Pacific theater of operations, an attack in which every member of his platoon, except him, died that day. He was left for dead. He did not remember his foot injury until, at age eighty-two, he started getting foot treatments for his Parkinson's disease. He'd *also* had no memory of the *attack* and the events of that horrific day until he started getting foot treatments. In this case, it would be impossible to say which came first: the psychological dissociation from the attack *or* the dissociation from his foot injury.

Then again, another patient had a history of unhealed childhood foot injury (detectable after he started getting treated for Parkinson's) but recalled becoming emotionally numb (dissociating from his heart) when he was an adult, in response to the tragic loss of his teenage daughter.

Curiously, we've found that a majority of our patients have a strong preference: they *want* their Parkinson's disease to be the result of a foot injury, and *not* the result of a feel-no-pain attitude. If they admit that they do have a feel-no-pain attitude, they would prefer that this attitude is the *result* of the foot injury. They usually don't want to consider that their foot injury failed to hurt and heal *because* they were able to, or maybe had already learned to, dissociate from their own pain.

Furthermore, they usually state, with firm conviction, that, if they had, after all, dissociated from their ability to feel their own physical and emotional pain, it wasn't their "fault." They "couldn't help it," because there had been negative forces at play in their lives.

Some of these patients want to talk for *hours* - hundreds of hours, if we'd let them – about the reasons that "forced" them to dissociate. They often insist that they have completely gotten over these "wrongs," and have moved on – but they keep talking about them. They sometimes get angry if one suggests that, so long as they continue to perceive them as "wrongs," they *haven't* gotten over them.

Based on our experience, this type of justification can make it harder for a person to get over his fears and move on. The patients who do succeed in overcoming a feel-no-pain attitude are the ones who quit blaming someone from the past, learn to be truly grateful for the problems of the past, and then focus primarily instead on correcting the attitudes with which they embrace the present.

Further addressing the point that most of our patients want their PD to have *only* a physical injury component and *no* psychological component, consider this: even in those cases where a pain-suppressing attitude and an unhealed foot injury are *both* present, the foot *injury*, per se, is never the "original" cause of the eventual development of Parkinson's. Again, the real problem is *not* that the person received a foot injury. Everyone gets foot injuries, but most people don't develop Parkinson's.

The real problem is that the injury never *healed*. Why didn't it heal? Because the person dissociated from the foot injury, so that it *couldn't* heal.

Even if the person in question was *not* dissociated from over-all ability to feel his body's physical and emotional pain, he *still* managed to dissociate from his foot injury.

In other words, *some degree of psychologically-induced denial always plays a role, whether the dissociation is directed at only a specific injury <u>or</u> at the prevention of feeling any and all physical or emotional pain.*

It might be body-wide dissociation from the heart that prevents one from feeling the foot injury. Or it might be a narrowly defined dissociation: dissociation from only a very specific foot injury. But these are both forms of *psychological* dissociation, and they both contribute to an electrical flow that eventually mimics that of *biological* dissociation.

In other words, there is always *some* form of psychological dissociation going on in Parkinson's disease. And the *long-term* result of this psychological dissociation, whether in the heart or the foot, is an electrical pattern that *matches* biological dissociation.

I'll be redundant here because many of our patients with Parkinson's have been highly resistant to understanding this: a foot injury, per se, does not cause Parkinson's. Again, nearly every human receives many foot injuries over the course of a lifetime, and they don't get Parkinson's disease. So it's not the fact of having had an injury that's at the root of the problem. The *dissociation* from the foot injury, and/or *dissociation* from the heart's ability to feel somatic pain, is at the root of the problem.

This brings us back to the reason for using FSR: the treatment must be extremely non-threatening – the goal of the treatment is to re-awaken the patient's awareness – after the patient has already decided, years earlier, that he doesn't want to have awareness - either in the injury area, or body-wide. We use FSR to help the patient get up the confidence to say to himself, "Even though I've been hurt, I'm finally safe, now – and actually, on some deeper level, I've always been safe, right along."

Time frame: variable. The injury itself is often easy enough to treat, requiring only a few weeks or months of treatment. The psychological component only heals when the person ceases to have the attitude that created it. This can take minutes, or it can take lifetimes.

3) Only a foot injury

And we've had patients who've dissociated from the foot injury, and *never* dissociated from their overall ability to feel their own physical and emotional pain.

Approximately five percent of our PD patients have manifested *no* generalized dissociation from the heart: the foot/ankle injury is an isolated event from which they have psychologically dissociated. With these patients, the Parkinson's is *usually* extremely easy to treat. In these cases, sometimes after only three or four hour-long, once a week FSR foot treatments, the foot injury begins to manifest, the bones or other displaced tissues slide back into place, the person relaxes internally, and the Parkinson's symptoms disappear like breath off a mirror.

As an aside, in our limited experience, five professional musicians with fairly early-stage Parkinson's have fallen into this category. I would guess that a profession like music, that requires a person to be guided by the cueings of his own heart in order to perform effectively, might not be interested in dissociating from physical or emotional pain, via shutting down the heart, even if he could. Or oppositely, a person who *has* shut down the input from the heart might have a hard time becoming a very successful musician.

To be sure, several of these musician patients had horrific, tragic life stories including violence and trauma, events that *could* have caused them to utterly turn off their hearts – and yet they had not.

How can one account for the differences in personal choices? I just don't know.

At any rate, we've treated professional, full-time working musicians, and all but one recovered in a matter of weeks. The one who continues to struggle with recovery had advanced Parkinson's when she started working with this program: she already needed assistance with basic activities of daily living. She also had more than just a foot injury: she definitely had steeled her heart due to childhood traumas, and yet had been a successful musician in spite of her dissociations.

As any neurologist can assure you, no two patients with Parkinson's are alike. The symptoms, the rate of progression, the sequence of symptoms, are different in every patient. This is a very personal, and personalized illness. It is impossible to give the "hard numbers," so dear to the heart of many people with Parkinson's, for how long the treatment will take. Still, for foot-only Parkinson's, we can say:

Time frame: fairly quick. A simple injury, with no other dissociations, might heal within a few weeks or months, at which time all symptoms of PD will cease.

Some case studies

A case of multiple injuries

Once in a while, even in patients without overall dissociation, a *secondary injury* needs to be addressed after the primary foot injury heals itself.

In one memorable case, after the foot injury healed, the patient, a professional musician, was still manifesting many Parkinson's symptoms, including tremor and rigidity in her face and arms, even though her *legs* had resumed normal, healthy movement. Like many of our other professional-musician PD patients, she had no attitudes characteristic of heart dissociation. She still seemed to have what you might call constant, "full-blown Parkinson's" in her upper body. This was very unlike those patients who slide into partial recovery after the foot injury has healed.

(Partial recovery is the name we use for patients whose symptoms are greatly reduced or gone after the foot injury heals, but who still tremor, or who slide now and then, or regularly, into full blown Parkinson's for a few hours or days at a time, when confronted with a "fearful" situation such as going to the in-laws – after which, the symptoms recede again until the next anxiety-inducing situation arises – which could be days, or *minutes*, later.)

A few years earlier, the above professional-musician patient had received a violent blow to the side of the head from a piece of falling furniture: she'd been unconscious for two days. Uncertain as to why her Parkinson's symptoms weren't completely clearing up now that her foot injury had healed, I decided to hold the area of the head injury. I had been firmly holding her utterly rigid temporal bones (near the ears). These bones, derived from ancestral gills, are supposed to perform a faint back and forth rotation with every incoming and outgoing breath. I'd been holding these bones, simply holding them with firm, supportive pressure, for around forty-five minutes when, suddenly, it felt to my hands as if all the bones in her skull were shifting around.

Right there in my office, she experienced the internal brain shift described in *Recovery from Parkinson's*. All her symptoms utterly ceased. The *internal* tremor, as well as the visible tremor, disappeared. Her neck relaxed, straightened out, and then, though her face had previously been a rigid mask, she smiled! And she announced, with utter certainty, "I'm all better!"

And she was.

That was more than ten years ago, and she's not had any Parkinson's symptoms since that day.

I shared the above case study to show that treating Parkinson's is not a simple matter of "fixing a foot." Every person with Parkinson's disease manifests his symptoms in a unique way. The sequence of the appearance of the symptoms and the symptoms themselves are different with each person. This is because each person with Parkinson's has a slightly different injury or collection of unhealed injuries. Each person with Parkinson's has his own level of dissociation mode-inducing behaviors, ranging from psychologically dissociating from a single injury, all the way to utter dissociation from the heart.

And yet, the same two treatment principles have been all that was necessary for *all* of our patients who've recovered. These principles are: 1) the injuries, if any, must heal, 2) the dissociation from somatic sensations of physical and emotional pain, if any, must cease.

When a patient does these two things, he recovers very, very quickly, from the symptoms of Parkinson's disease.

Two case studies illustrating refusal to deal with fear of pain

Some patients have such a dread fear of experiencing the sensations of their own physical and emotional pain that they are uninterested in changing their "dissociation from the heart."

One such patient told me, "The *whole point* of life is to not feel pain!" She was adamant that her refusal to feel pain was more important than recovering from Parkinson's. She was determined to *not* be able to feel her physical body despite understanding the problems that her mental numbness was causing her. She insistently instructed us, "Just hold my foot and I'll get better!"

Needless to say, she did not recover even though our team, and others, held her unhealed foot and hip injuries for many, many sessions.

Another patient, tremoring violently and barely able to move, was very proud of his inability to feel pain: it was his greatest accomplishment. He bragged that when his wife left him, he had felt absolutely no pain. He'd been married three times; all three wives had left him in their turn, and he was *proud* that he never felt anything – no emotion, no pain – at any of those three times.

When I suggested that he might benefit from learning how to feel, and how to correctly deal with pain, he proudly whispered to me with what was left of his voice, "I'm wealthy, I'm a huge success! And you're only a doctor, paid by the hour!" His violent tremoring continued, his body was rigidly contorted into almost a fetal posture as he continued to whisper, "and it's my refusal to feel pain that's made me what I am today!"

I wholeheartedly agreed with him.

The strangest case studies of all

Finally, to make it even more interesting, some people – even some with injuries - have abruptly recovered from Parkinson's without having their injuries treated in any way.

Some have been aware of our research; some have not. Their commonality is that, after struggling with the symptoms of Parkinson's disease, either for a short while or for many years, they have made a decision to turn *all* control of their heart and their lives over to a higher power. By doing so, they have necessarily abandoned their "ability" to be numb to their own pain.

In the few cases of this type of which I am aware, a patient has "surrendered" to a higher power. Gratefully choosing to *embrace* the illness as a learning experience and gift from God, while deciding to devote one's life to finding a closer, more "feeling-the-presence" relationship with the Divine despite the illness, he has opted for devotion to a higher power *as opposed to* struggling to overcome the Parkinson's. And then, unexpectedly, he has experienced nearly instantaneous recovery.

In some cases, the Parkinson' symptoms simply went away. In other cases, the Parkinson's symptoms went away *and* the person suddenly became highly aware of extreme pain in the foot or ankle, from a long-forgotten injury. The pain of the injury might have been extreme, but because this person allowed the pain to be solaced in the protective love of the newly feel-able higher power, the pain was perceived as *only* "breath-taking," or even "fascinating," but *not* terrifying.

In other words, despite the pain, the person was able to say, "I'm safe now – in spite of the current pain" and then *experience* the pain, and the subsequent, natural healing of the injury, without fear.

This latter situation was the case in my own unexpected recovery from all the classic symptoms of Parkinson's disease.

Because these cases do not involve any physical treatment of the injuries, they suggest that the psychological change, "the surrender," and the concomitant "willingness to *feel*" might be more important than the foot therapy.

For many people with Parkinson's, devotional surrender and willingness to feel often seem like two unrelated concepts: the first seems to require "giving up hope" or "quitting" and the second usually can't even be imagined.

But people who have given their hearts over to a higher power have quickly realized that the primary way one communicates with that higher power is by *feeling* its presence in the heart. Surrender, in these cases, does *not* mean giving up hope. It merely means paying attention to and obeying the sensations that occur in the heart, instead of the fear-based instructions coming from the head. In "surrender to a higher power," the ego surrenders to the heart.

In a case when a person with Parkinson's utterly surrenders, he abandons his personal desires and life preferences in trade for personal communion with Love, God, The Divine, or whatever he calls that Energy and Wisdom that creates our very atoms and holds them together. When he does this, all his *fear*-based electrical disarray will instantaneously cease. After all, all fears are desire-based: for example, "I don't *want* to die," "I don't *want* to be made fun of," and "I don't *want* to feel pain" are the building blocks on which we decide to *fear* death, mockery, or pain. We fear them because they run counter to our ego-based desires.

When he lets go of these desires, or "surrenders" them, the fear-based signals and dissociation-type signals in his heart can cease. He automatically switches over to parasympathetic-type signals. The only electrical disarrays remaining in the body will be those kept in place by unhealed injuries, scars, or other ongoing illness. When the heart is completely uninhibited by the mind (parasympathetic mode) and open to feeling everything in the body, any unhealed injuries will necessarily become truly and completely *felt* in the heart – by virtue of their electrical disarray. And once the injuries are *felt*, this information can be transmitted to the brain and acknowledged *without* fear, as per the instructions from the heart. Then, the injury can begin to heal.

The body is designed to heal. When it *doesn't* heal, it's because the mind or some pathological electrical presentation, either externally or internally induced, is doing something to prevent it from so doing.

In cases of spontaneous healing from Parkinson's via surrender, a person may still have to work out his foot injury. But it won't be problematic, even if it is painful: it will heal, just as it is supposed to do. Help may be beneficial in these cases: if the leg was broken, now might be the time to get it encased in a cast. If the ankle was twisted, now might be the time to get it gently held, or wrap it in an elastic bandage, for temporary support. In other words, the injury transitions to an "ordinary" injury that will be able to heal if given normal, appropriate support.

Why we use Yin Tui Na

Recovering using *only* "surrendering one's entire life to a high power" is very difficult to do. It is usually easier for a person to surrender his dissociation by small steps. Using FSR or other types of Yin Tui Na, such as highly modified (much more passive) craniosacral therapy, a patient can learn, first, to surrender control over his injury. After surrendering control over the injury, he is on his way to, hopefully, surrendering his heart dissociations (if any) that he uses to control his ability to not feel pain.

Also, some people struggle mightily to overcome their doctor's fiat that Parkinson's is incurable. When they begin to experience the earliest recovery symptoms, the ones that come about from the cessation of injury – via FSR – even if they only experience *partial* recovery due to their continuing dissociation from their heart, their confidence nevertheless increases. They begin to see that, just maybe, the doctor was wrong.

In many cases, following treatment and healing of the injury with FSR, the only remaining symptom is tremor. The confidence gained by seeing the cessation of rigidity – or the resumption of rigidity only during times of fear – can serve as stepping stone towards overcoming the heart dissociation and fear of feeling pain that still holds the tremor in place.

People with Parkinson's tend to be *very* susceptible to suggestion: the placebo effect. In our limited experience, they usually are *adamant* that they are *not* susceptible to placebo effect, but excellent research shows that they very much are. They are particularly susceptible to their own negative thoughts. They are also highly influenced by their doctors' proclamation of incurability.

Overcoming these two negative factors can be easier if the patient sees that he is experiencing some symptoms of recovery, even if he is not yet completely recovered. And so, even though, in a perfect world, we might be able to just say to a PD patient, "Just stop dissociating from your ability to feel!" this is not practical in the real world. Therefore, we use FSR to focus on the injuries, if any, to *start* the patient down the path of recovery.

As an aside, when a doctor says an illness is incurable, he only means that *he* doesn't have the cure. *Every* so-called incurable illness has examples of people recovering – they just recovered in a manner that the doctor cannot explain.[1]

And so we promote the use of Yin Tui Na techniques such as Forceless, Spontaneous Release, (FSR), for people who plan to recover from Parkinson's disease. Yes, a person might be able to recover on his own, "simply" by surrendering control over his heart to a higher power or using whatever means necessary to end his self-induced dissociation from his injury and/or his heart. And yes, when the dissociation stops, the physical injuries will manifest, and then heal on their own.

But because many patients have been able to completely recover or at least partially recover by starting off on the easier path of using a form of supportive holding that brings one's attention to a dissociated injury, we continue to promote this form of therapy for people with Parkinson's disease.

Not so surprisingly, considering their fear level, many people with Parkinson's do not want any help from another person on their road to recovery. A common battle cry is, "I'd rather do it myself." (Translation: I don't trust anyone enough to let him mess with me; I'm afraid of the damage that the "wrong" person might do.) We get many, many emails asking, "Can't I just do FSR on myself?" and even "Won't it be *better* if I do the FSR on myself?" Many people want to do FSR on themselves because they don't want anyone to know that they have Parkinson's – an imperfection.

I must admit, we've heard from two people who did the FSR on their own feet, and recovered from Parkinson's. But they performed the work on themselves because they genuinely could not find anyone to do the work on them. They were not trying to be secretive or self-contained wonders.

We know of another person who was able to re-associate with the heart and with the foot injury, and heal it, by doing a Chinese technique of Qi Gong – mental manipulation of channel Qi. However, *most* people with Parkinson's who do Qi Gong are *not* able to access body parts from which they've dissociated: we've had Parkinson's patients who were long-time Qi Gong teachers or were yoga teachers (yoga is another art in which a person is

---

[1] For example, schizophrenia is considered an incurable illness: doctors are unable to cure it. And yet, a study that followed up on people who'd been diagnosed with schizophrenia found that many years after their diagnosis, 25% of them had recovered. Despite this very significant number, schizophrenia is still considered incurable because the *doctors* are unable to cure it. You can read about this in *A Beautiful Mind,* by Sylvia Nasar. She tells the story of a Nobel laureate, John Forbes Nash, who conquered his "incurable" schizophrenia.

In the same way, MDs often say that the common cold has no cure. Happily, in Asian medicine, the common cold is one of the easiest things to treat. As my widely esteemed teacher, Dr. Jeffery Pang, when confronted with this western-medicine "truth," used to say with genuine puzzlement, "Who would ever go to a doctor that can't even cure a common cold?"

supposed to focus on the energy in the body). Despite long-term participation in energy-control techniques, they never even *detected* their unhealed injuries or heart dissociation.

In general, a person who is determined that he doesn't *want* "someone else's help," a person who "only wants to recover on my own, own my own terms," will probably *not* recover. The stubborn attitude of "I'd rather do it myself" is the opposite of surrender: this determination to go it alone is the same as demanding that one's own will (ego) must be in charge. This is very similar to demanding control over how much pain one feels. Sometimes, the *best thing* a person with Parkinson's can do is admit that he will benefit from the ministrations of another human or a higher power; admit that he cannot overcome his physical problems and his psychological dissociations by himself.

If a person is afraid of being helped by others – a not uncommon sentiment among people with Parkinson's – non-invasive, patient, supportive FSR might be a crucial part of overcoming this particular fear. It can almost be a leap of faith – the beginnings of surrender – for a PD patient to allow himself to be worked on by some imperfect human who might do an imperfect job.

In summary, how many treatments will it take before a person's injuries begin to heal? There is no way to know. Every patient is different.

How many days, months, or years will it take before a person decides to stop dissociating from his heart? There is no way to know. It's a moment-to-moment *choice*, not a cumulative process. Every patient is different.

What is the time-range? From several weeks, to many years, to many lifetimes. Every patient is different.[1]

One thing is certain: the many patients who have affirmed to me that their *own* case is going to take a *long* time on the road to recovery have been absolutely right.

But this much is also certain: the immortal soul does not have idiopathic Parkinson's disease. *Someday*, in this life or in some other, the person with Parkinson's *will* eventually learn how to *correctly* deal with pain. He will stop dissociating from it and experience it maturely, fearlessly, with gratitude for the bigger picture.

When that happens, he will no longer choose to employ the mental techniques that can lead to Parkinson's.

---

[1] I've had patients say to me that they feel they've had Parkinson's before, that the whole scenario feels so familiar, as if they have played it out many times before. One patient, upon being diagnosed, spontaneously exclaimed, "Not again!"

Chapter three

Forceless, Spontaneous Release: a *very* Yin type of Yin Tui Na

Tui Na is sometimes translated as "massage." It would be better to translate it as "therapeutic body work."

Yin Tui Na is a phrase that refers to any of the "light touch" or seemingly passive forms of hands-on bodywork. For example, gentle craniosacral work is a Yin form of Tui Na. This type of work is usually thought of as non-invasive, or minimalistic.

Oppositely, *Yang* Tui Na refers to vigorous or highly manipulative forms of body work. For example, the intense manipulations of Rolfing or the bone-cracking types of chiropractic work are both Yang forms of Tui Na.

One of the *most* passive forms of Yin Tui Na is Forceless, Spontaneous Release, or FSR. You might think of it as a *very* minimalistic type of Yin Tui Na. It's useful in treating areas that are painful because of tension from injury or fear. And yet, when treating people with an injury from which they have *dissociated*, and in our experience this includes most people with Parkinson's disease, we use an even more minimalistic variant of FSR: we just get comfy and then sit in one place, holding the patient for as long as it takes.

This chapter will first discuss the basic technique of FSR, and then cover the "just sit there" variant that is used with people who've dissociated from their pain.

Basic FSR

The technique of Forceless, Spontaneous Release, FSR, is extremely simple. It consists of firmly holding a body part between two hands in such a snug way that, soon, the patient's *body part* doesn't really notice that it is being held.

In response to the support, the body part relaxes. It resumes the electrical patterns of parasympathetic mode: the healing mode.

Then again, if, after a minute or two, there is no relaxation response, a tiny nudge, quickly bringing the hands ever-so-slightly close together, and then letting the hands spring back to their original position, will usually evoke a relaxation response.

The relaxation

The whole point of the strong, supportive holding is that it allows the patient to relax in the part of his body that is being held.

You, the practitioner, are not *imposing* relaxation on the patient. You are just providing utter support.

And if the patient is physically and emotionally able to bring awareness into the area that you are holding, then when that part of the patient's body is held snugly enough, that area will spontaneously relax, letting go of retained tension.

If there is no response

If the area does not respond to supportive holding, but remains rigid and unmoved, you need to suspect that you are dealing with a body part that is either holding a temporary *high* level of tension due to pain or recent injury, or it is an area from which the patient has dissociated.

Temporary high levels of tension can also occur if the patient is nervous, doesn't trust the practitioner, or is dealing with some other emotional shock at the present time, and is somewhat "locked down."

If there is a response

Try doing a bit of holding on a *healthy* practice partner. When working on a healthy practice partner, the body part being held will very likely respond to your holding by relaxing. The relaxation demonstrates that the body area you just "worked on" is *capable* of responding. If the area is *capable* of quickly responding (relaxing), you can know that you are *not* working with an area that is frozen in place by some pain, stress, or dissociative pattern.

Then again, sometimes there is a *bit* of tension in the area that you are holding. The body part that you are holding might not move right at first, but might relax after a few moments, or a few minutes.

This tension might have been related to an old injury that has not *completely* healed. In such a case, the physical body might not have completed its healing. Or in other cases, the body may have completed its healing, but the emotions from the injury might still be keeping tension in the area. However, your holding, if done correctly, may *soon* evoke a relaxation response in the patient.

If there is unfinished physical healing to be done, the relaxation can give the "all clear" sign to the brain, so that the physical healing will be completed. Or, this relaxation can remove the last of the emotional tension, if any.

Your hands move when the patient responds

Your hands can detect the patient's relaxation. Usually, your hands will physically move – change away from your starting hand positions – because of the patient's relaxation. When the patient's body part relaxes, your hands – sticking closely to the patient – will have followed the relaxation movements of the patient and thus moved away from their original position. You can feel this movement in your hands. Often, the relaxation causes enough movement in the patient's muscles that the movement in your own hands is *visually* obvious.

How long do you hold?

How long do you leave your hands in place? Until there is movement in the part of the patient's body that is being held, followed by a static shift that repulses your hands.

When I say that "your hands will have moved," I am allowing for a wide range of possibilities. Sometimes, the relaxation response is very small. Your hands might just travel a fraction of an inch: a "flinch" type of response. Even so, you will have noticed that you weren't holding a piece of wood. There *was* a small response.

Oppositely, sometimes you might need to clamp on securely as the patient's skin responds by moving back and forth, or twisting, or making fairly large movements. It is not unusual for the practitioner to place his hands firmly and securely on the patient, with one hand, say, on the *top* of the arm and the other hand opposite, on the *bottom*, only to find himself, moments later, with one of his hands on the *left* side of the patient's arm and his other hand on the *right* side: left and right, rather than top and bottom.

The patient's muscles will have responded to the support by relaxing in such a way that the practitioner's hands have moved, sometimes *visibly* moved, away from the starting point.

If the patient's body part moved, it means that the body part is *capable* of relaxing. If the body part does *not* move, even after several seconds, it means that a holding pattern, some kind of tension, is prevailing in the area being supported. In order to treat the tension, or holding pattern, the health practitioner simply continues to support the area for another five to ten minutes, or however long it takes for the area to relax. Typically, the non-responsiveness in the area will "let go" (release) within a few minutes. If it's taking more than a few minutes, tiny nudges of the area will often provoke a release.

Visually undetectable, sometimes purely mental, nudges in one direction or another may be performed, if necessary, to determine whether or not the area being held is capable of reflexively responding to either the support or the minute suggestions of movement.

The hands are removed after the body part being held *relaxes or otherwise responds in some way*. The treatment, in *that particular* body part, is then finished. Very likely, you will continue the treatment with a nearby area, until you have confirmed that the whole vicinity of the injured area relaxes or shows some sort of response, quickly, in answer to your holding.

The relaxation, also known as the release of the holding pattern, allows any twisting or displacement in the bones or soft tissue to unwind themselves or slide back into the correct locations. These actions do not need to be *guided* by the health practitioner. The patient's body knows exactly where any displaced tissues need to go, and will take care of this – as soon as the holding pattern ceases.

This technique can help with almost any sort of displacement injury and pain. The technique is simultaneously a diagnostic procedure and a treatment protocol. If the area being held is not responsive, we can make a diagnosis: there is a holding pattern in this location. Then, to treat the holding pattern, we simply continue holding, or maybe do some imperceptible nudging, until the holding pattern lets go.

The variation of basic FSR that is used for dissociation

When working with a person with Parkinson's, we do the usual FSR holding, following the relaxation movement with our hands, and letting go after a static release – but it all happens in slow motion, compared to using FSR on most other patients. It may take several sessions before the patient feels safe while being held – you may need to start working on the patient's foot by holding the patient's upper leg, or even arm, at least until he learns to trust you. It may take many sessions, even months, or years, before the injured area relaxes. After it does relax, and the tension is released, the injured area may want the supportive hands to stay in place for hours, rather than minutes, before it gives a static shift that signals "You can go away, I'm OK after all."

In other words, the entire process is the same, but the time frames might be much longer. The practitioner needs to be prepared for extended periods of non-invasive support.

Also, the thoughts of the practitioner must be even *less* invasive than during "usual" FSR. The practitioner's mind *must* be minding its own business: it should *not* be focused on the injury.

The treatment should be less physically invasive, as well. This means less, or no, subtle nudging of the stuck area to see if the tension can be jostled loose, at first. Even giving a mental nudge to an area might be perceived, during the first few sessions, as too invasive.

Of course, even with healthy people, the response will come faster if the practitioner is not trying to impose any sort of mental expectation on the patient. But Parkinson's patients tend to be actively wary of the possibility that the practitioner might try to impose some sort of thoughts, "wrong energy," or even worse, value judgments, on them. So when treating people with Parkinson's, the practitioner wants his hands to be providing firm support, and his mind to be somewhere else *entirely* – maybe putting together a shopping list for groceries.[1]

When treating people with Parkinson's, or anyone who has dissociated from an unhealed injury, the diagnostic principle is the same as for painful injuries and tension: if nothing moves in response to touch, there is a holding pattern in place. But in dissociation cases, the *reason* for the immobility is different. The body is not just using tension to protect the injured area: the mind is actively *denying the existence* of the injury. This dissociation causes a marked, and sometimes long-lasting, lack of response to FSR in the area being held. This means that the treatment might take much longer than with a normal injury.

Although a *healthy* person might manifest a response to hands-on support within the blink of an eye, and a person with a painful injury might only respond after being held for several minutes, or even ten minutes, before letting go of the holding pattern, people with Parkinson's are in a class of their own. They might not respond to this type of holding for hours, weeks, even months.

And in the beginning, even the tiniest of nudges might cause the person with Parkinson's disease to tighten up in the injured area, instead of relaxing. So when treating people with Parkinson's, or anyone with an injury from which they've dissociated, we just hold the injured area. And hold it. And hold it.

Eventually, even in a person with Parkinson's disease, when the person's body part that's being held begins to relax, the patient's awareness of that body part is also becoming involved. If the patient is able to become aware of that body part while in a relaxed

---

[1] Correct intention on the part of the practitioner can be very important. When treating most people with Parkinson's, the "correct intention" should be "Mind my own business." It is nice if your "own business" has to do with keeping your mind on something uplifting, but the point is, do not impose your issues, even your good intentions, on the patient.

I remember one classroom student saying, "I feel like I'm not getting anywhere with this patient. I'm praying for Mother Teresa of Calcutta to inspire him and help him, but I just don't know...he's *so* rigid..."

I suggested that she forget about the patient and ask Mother Teresa to help her, the student, with her *own* problems. She did so, and within moments, she said, "Oh. I see. The patient's skin doesn't seem to be fighting me anymore."

I have often beheld beneficial changes in very "stubborn" patients while my mind was on highly mundane matters, such as compiling a grocery list. As for the idea of "correct intention," it might best be understood, in the Parkinson's context, as "don't let your thoughts wander into negative areas, and keep your thoughts on something that is uplifting for *you*."

(parasympathetic) manner, then the holding patterns and tensions can begin to release. Eventually, the body part being held relaxes enough that the components in the injured area start to move and realign themselves.

When this happens, and we see and/or feel our own hands being moved as we maintain close contact, we can say, "The patient has released the holding pattern" or "The patient has started fixing himself."
We don't say, "*I* fixed the patient."

When the Parkinson's patient's rigid body parts do start to move, it's because the patient's attention, his subconscious attention, the part of his mind that regulates subconscious protection of the injury, has been brought to bear on the injury – and has decided that things are *safe enough* that he can start to notice what's going on in the injured area.
It seems as if the FSR's snugness and the non-moving, firm support, like that of a human ace bandage, over a long time, is the thing that suggests, "Now I am safe!"

How long will it take? It's impossible to predict.

So when working with a Parkinson's patient, or anyone who has dissociated from an injury, settle yourself into as comfortable a position as possible: keep your spine straight, shoulders relaxed, and feet well planted on the floor. Be prepared to sit for a *long* time without moving. Then, firmly place your hands on either side of the unresponsive area, supporting it, the same as one would do with any FSR treatment. Then, settle in for the long haul. Keep the hands as snug as possible while they remain fairly motionless for as long as necessary (usually the length of the treatment session), while actively working to keep your mind uninvolved with whatever the patient's injury might be doing.

Chapter four

FSR technique: setting your hands on the patient

FSR technique might be broken down into four steps: 1) setting your hands on the patient, 2) following the patient's ensuing relaxation movements with your hands, 3) diagnostically making use of relaxation responses, if any, and 4) letting go.

This chapter and the three following chapters are devoted to these four steps.

Positioning the hands

With you and your practice partner sitting down, place the palm side of your hand flush against some part of the forearm of your partner. Then place your other hand on the opposite side of the forearm. (See fig. 4.1.)

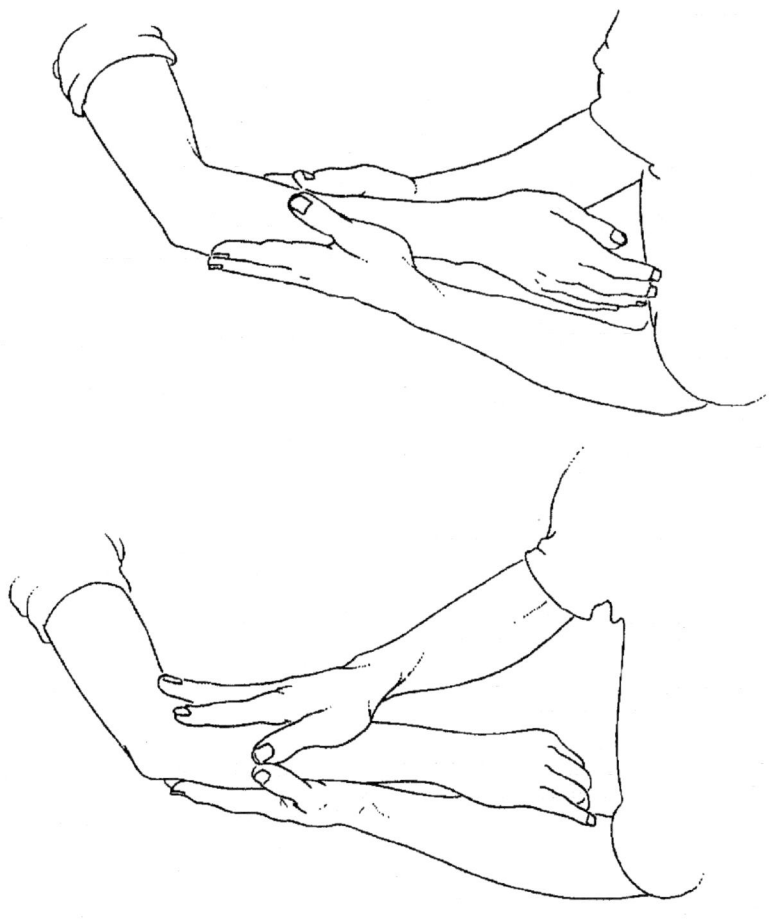

Fig. 4.1
Two examples of placing your hands on opposite sides of a body part

It does not matter exactly where your hands are. The important thing is that your two hands are more or less opposite each other.

Your own physical comfort is important. Position your chair so that you are comfortable.

If your patient or practice partner has an injury in the area you are holding, you may need to sit fairly still for several minutes. If you are working on a Parkinson's patient, you may be sitting in one position, barely moving, for an hour. So your ability to get comfortable and stay relaxed is more important than the exact placement of your hands.

Slumping back in a soft chair may seem like a comfortable way to sit, but this type of "comfortable" is not easy to maintain for very long. You will be able to work longer and better if you can learn to sit upright, with good posture, while your arms suspend softly from the shoulder. Your wrists should be relaxed – able to move or flex in response to the patient's movements.

Although most *Parkinson's* treatments will begin on the leg, it's easiest for the beginner to practice FSR on a partner's arm. No physiological reason – it's just that arms are far easier to access: you can both be sitting in chairs when you work on arms. When you work on legs, the subject usually needs to be lying down.

Asking permission

Before grabbing your practice partner's arm or leg, ask permission to hold the arm or leg.

After getting comfortably settled into your work chair or stool, with the patient sitting in a chair or lying down on the treatment table with his shoes off, ask, "May I hold your arm?" or "May I hold your leg?"

Ask permission every time you begin to work on a patient. This simple question becomes rather ceremonial. It is a very polite way of honoring the patient's autonomy. You aren't just going to wait until your patient looks comfortable and then grab for his arm or leg. You ask permission to hold, and then after the patient says, "Yes," you start.

This may seem very formal and unnecessary, but you will see very quickly that patients learn to anticipate this little bit of courtesy and respond pleasantly.

Of course, the first time you work on a patient and ask this, they may reply, "Of course! That's what I'm here for!" But after a few sessions, they will understand that they are participating in a respectful formality, and they usually learn to enjoy it.

Use your palms

The *palms* of your hands are the main contact point. Do not try to hold the patient with your fingers. Your fingers can of course be making contact, as well, but the center of the strength of your holding comes from the center of the palms of your hands.

When we hold something with our fingers, our fingers curve inward (flexed), which is to say, with the fingers moving towards the "fist" position. Notice in the illustrations that opened this chapter how the fingers are the opposite of flexed – they are slightly extended. In terms of muscle movements, "extended" means the opposite direction of "flexed." This finger extension is not always necessary, but sometimes, depending on the curve of the patient's skin, the fingers need to be relaxed enough that they assume an extended position in order to get the center of the palm of the hand firmly connected to the patient.

Of course, there will be times when the palm of the hand doesn't fit easily. For example, when holding the arch of the foot, you will place one hand over the top of the foot – directly over the arch area (the "saddle" of the foot) – and the other hand on the sole of the foot, *under* the arch. But, if the size and angles of the arch prevent the *palm* of your hand from getting solid, flat contact on the sole of the arch, you might use the *back* of your hand, instead of the palm of your hand, to provide firm support to the sole of the foot in the arch area. The firm contact over the widest possible area is the main thing – *not* the electrical properties contained in the palm of the hand.

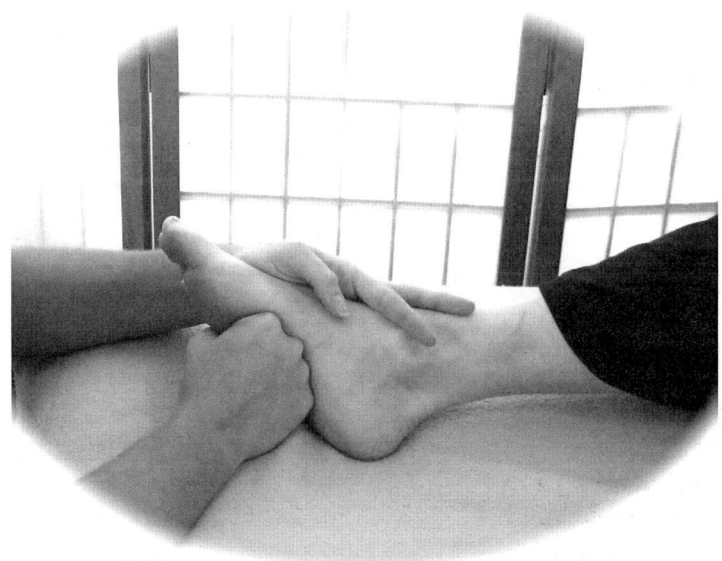

Fig. 4.2 Using the back of the hand to make firm contact with the sole of the foot

You should *not* grip with your fingers just because you're working on an area that is hard to access with your palm; you should find some way to make firm contact with some part of your hand that will maximize the sensation that the patient's body is being held in place with an ace bandage (also known as an elastic bandage) – but *not* held in place with vice grips.

Pressure

The amount of pressure that your hands exert on the partner is *very important*. You should make firm, fairly complete skin-to-skin (even if there is clothing in between) contact. The goal is to hold the patient with such complete support that, very soon, he cannot feel your hands.

Because the completeness of the support is more important than the exact, precise location of where you are holding, it is important that you find a way to nestle your hands into the contours of your partner's body part, even if such a holding position is not exactly the location of holding that you originally had in mind. When you have gotten your hands nestled into a place that feels comfy and "settled in", your partner, curiously enough, will often volunteer that you have put your hands in "just the right place."

Now let's back up a bit and look more closely at what you are doing, looking at one hand at a time. Let's assume in the following explanation that you are putting one hand on the upper side of your patient's arm, and your other hand underneath his arm. In actual practice, of course, one hand might be on the left side and the other on the right side. But for clarity, let's assume that your hands are on the "top" (closer to the ceiling) and "bottom" (closer to the floor) of the patient's arm.

Upper hand

If you are sitting in a comfortable position, you will be able to let your upper hand drop gently from your shoulder and come to rest on the patient. Your hand should be resting like a dead weight, with the full weight of your hand plopped down on your partner. Now, add just a bit *more* pressure – enough so that the patient's skin isn't possibly going to slip out from under your hand. You should be using a fair amount of force, by the way. If you are using *any* muscles to *prevent* your hand from pushing too hard onto your partner, you are holding too lightly. Use gravity, and then a bit more.

If you aren't sure what I mean by "dead weight" and then a little more, you might want to abandon your partner for a moment and try this practice exercise: sit in an armless chair. Let your hand flop down onto your thigh. Let your hand just sit there, held in place by gravity. Notice that your hand isn't making complete contact with your leg: there's a gap on the palm of the hand where air is present. Now, leave your hand in place and lean forward just a few inches so that your hand is supporting the weight of your torso. Notice that your hand is now making firm contact with your leg. It's not that you are trying to push *against* your leg. It's more that the weight of your torso is causing your hand to make a very *complete* contact with your leg. The force needed to make a complete contact is the exact right amount of pressure to use in FSR.

Again, *don't* push your hand hard into your thigh as if you were trying to leave an imprint of your hand: that would be too much pressure. Don't rest your hand gingerly, as if your thighs were sunburned: that would be not enough pressure. Let your shoulders relax and sag down. Let your hand rest heavily on your thigh while supporting your slightly forward body. That is the exact correct amount of pressure for your top hand. Now, take this hand off your thigh and respectfully allow it to plop back down with the same degree of weight onto your practice partner's arm.

Lower hand

Use the exact same amount of pressure with the lower hand that you use with the upper hand.

If you want, you can abandon your partner again for a moment and practice holding your thigh again, but this time you will use both hands. Let your first hand flop down onto one side of your thigh, and place your other hand on the opposite side of your thigh. Lean your torso forward just a bit so that the hands must make a more complete contact in order to stay where they are.

Another image: imagine that your thigh is a mound of bread dough. Use as much pressure between the hands as you would need to use to keep the lifeless bread dough from dropping to the ground. Do not hold the limp "bread dough" gingerly and do not hold it with your fingertips. You might even spread your fingers apart so that you can get the centers of your palms as close to the "bread dough" as possible. The fingers might be slightly flexed or slightly extended – whatever position best enables you to have the palms of your hands as firmly connecting to the thigh as possible. Have a firm grip on the two sides of the "bread dough" of your thigh, but don't be leaving imprints of your hands or fingers in your flesh. Just hold it enough so that even if the thigh goes completely limp, it won't fall to the floor.

The point that your hands need to be making to the patient is this: even if your muscles in this area were to become as limp as bread dough, I am giving you enough support so that you won't fall to the floor.

In other words, I've got you, you are safe, you may become as limp as bread dough, if you want, and no harm will come to you.

Try placing both hands on your partner's forearm again, using the same amount of support that you used to support your thigh when you imagined it was as limp as bread dough.

Always use two hands

When your hands are on either side of the patient's body part, your two hands should be pressing on *each other* with the necessary amount of force.

You *never* press down on the patient's body part with just one hand. If you do this, the patient will automatically use energy to push back against your hand. When you are "holding" the patient, the pressure you are using is NOT pressure being applied to the patient – your two hands are applying equal pressure against *each other*. By supporting the patient with *two* hands, and the two hands are pressing against *each other*, the patient doesn't need to "push back" against anything. The patient is being supported. The two hands are pushing firmly on *each other*, not on the patient.

When you are holding the patient, what you should really be doing is pressing your hands together. It just so happens that a patient's body part is in between your hands. Ignore the patient's body part. If you want to focus on anything, focus on how your two hands are pressing on each other even though something has come between them.

When your focus is on your two hands applying firm pressure on each other, and you are ignoring the body part that is resting between your hands, you will be feeling what it's like to provide firm, supportive holding.

Eventually, you will be able to notice all sorts of things going on in the patient's body part, while keeping your primary focus on your own hands.

You will then be able to notice subtle changes or tensions in the patient's body part, and you can then use this information to modify the exact placement of your hands, or the exact amount of pressure that you are using, so as to help the patient relax even more. These modifications will be almost automatic, even reflexive. They will occur in response to what the patient's body is silently telling you. Don't worry about what your hands will do at this point – they will be working with the patient on their own, without your mind getting involved.

Much as a good dairy farmer intuitively knows how to touch each of his cows to keep them calm, at some point your *hands* will know just how much pressure to use in response to each of your patient's body's signals, even if you don't consciously know how much pressure is needed.

How much pressure to use – yet again

"How much pressure?" is the most frequently asked question.

I repeat, you should use as much force as you need to make the patient feel perfectly supported. If the effect of gravity should suddenly stop working on the patient's body part, your pressure would continue to hold the patient in the same place.

All of us maintain a certain amount of unconscious pressure in our muscles – at least enough to combat gravity, and to combat the pressure from the air around us.

If you are holding with at least the force of gravity, the patient will be able to stop unconsciously fighting the force of gravity in that particular body part. This unconscious work of combating gravity (on the part of the patient) can cease. The part of the patient's body that you are holding can relax much more deeply than usual.

Oddly enough, when you provide just enough support, supplanting all the pressure the patient was maintaining to combat gravity, air pressure, and anticipation of needing to move, the patient's body soon will be *unable* to tell that you are applying any force at all. The patient will feel as if, for all intents and purposes, your hands are not even there.

Have you ever swaddled a crying baby? Swaddling blankets are wrapped so snugly around a baby that he can't even move – not at all. And when the baby is swaddled snugly enough, he is able to relax. When he is so constrained by the tight blanket that he *can't* move his own muscles, when he doesn't *need* to move his own muscles to combat the strange, heavy world that is such a contrast to his previous, weightless world in utero, he relaxes as if he was once again floating and weightless.

When ranchers need to calm a frightened calf, they usher him into a "squeezer," or "press," a simple device consisting of boards on both flanks of the calf. A rope pulls the two sides of the press together, squeezing the cow until he can't move. When the calf feels sufficient support, he relaxes. His muscles, being supported by the press, don't need to maintain any tension of their own. The calf calms down both physically and mentally.

The principles of swaddling and pressing are the same principles used in Yin Tui Na: solid, unyielding support applied to a patient in a particular body area can physically and mentally relax that body area.

Don't be "gentle"

Do not hold gently; nothing can be more annoying. Resting your hands or fingertips ever so lightly on a patient is a sure way to either tickle or irritate him.

Hold the body part with such support that even if the table on which your partner's body is resting was to be pulled away, your holding would prevent his body from falling to the floor.

Don't manipulate

Don't try to physically *or even mentally* manipulate the limb you are holding. At this stage, when you are practicing how to hold without either insufficient or excessive physical or mental pressure, consider that any intention on your part, even for the good of the patient, is a form of psychological manipulation. So don't be imagining any particular outcome as a result of your support. Have *no* intention in mind for how the practice partner should respond.

Pressure without intention: the harried mother example

The following example illustrates what I mean by solid support without intention.

Picture the scene: a harried mother is trying to cook dinner. She is standing at the stove, stirring food in two pots. One pot has almost come to a boil and needs to be watched closely. The other pot is bubbling away and needs frequent stirring. Just out of arm's reach, her four-year old child is pestering her two-year old child. The younger child is just starting to scream in frustration. The mother cannot reach them because she is stirring the dinner, plus she is talking to her friend on the phone; the phone is the old fashioned kind, attached by a cord to the wall.

She is not using her hand to hold the phone, the phone is cradled between her ear and her raised shoulder. She is alternating between telling the youngsters to stop fighting and trying to arrange a babysitting swap with her friend for tomorrow.

Meanwhile, she is also holding a baby on her hip. It is not her *own* baby; she is babysitting for another neighbor, who should be home shortly. The mother has the neighbor's baby wedged up against her left hip and she has her left arm wrapped around the baby. Baby is stuck between the firm left hip and the snug left arm. Baby is in *solid*. Baby is going *nowhere*.

With her right arm, mother is now alternating between adding some spice to the dinner and tasting it. Mother is still listening to her friend on the phone and is stage-whispering to the older child a command to stop hitting the younger child with the stuffed weasel.

Here is my question: who is the most contented person in the room?

If you guessed the neighbor's baby, you are absolutely right. The baby is looking around, taking it all in, reveling in the fact that he doesn't have any social interactions going on. Baby is being held so closely that he can't move. With this level of firm support, baby doesn't even notice that he is being held. Baby has such complete trust in that firm support coming from the hip and the embracing arm that baby does not notice the pressure from the mother's hip and arm. Also, and most importantly, *the mother is not paying any attention to the baby* with her eyes or words. The baby is physically relaxed and comfortable.

Of course, when the baby's mother returns, baby will probably go into his regular routine of crying or cooing at his own mother, doing all the things it has already learned to do to fulfill his mother's expectations. But while the baby is being held tightly on the busy mother's hip with no one looking at him, no one cooing at him, no one expecting anything of him, being *completely ignored*, he is able to take it all in with wide-eyed wonder, amusement or contentment, and his body will be physically at peace.

How is the above mother holding the baby? Snugly! That's the way you hold a person with Parkinson's disease.

Comfort for the practitioner

In the example above, the mother is doing whatever she needs to do to be comfortable. No doubt she has one hip swung way out to the side to support the baby. This isn't an example of "good posture," but by having one hip out to the side as a seat for the baby, the mother is able to be very comfortable while holding that extra weight.

What with gravity, the mother's hip, *and* the additional, very firm lateral support provided by the left arm, the baby is nice and snug.

The amount of pressure you should use is the same as the mother is using on the baby: enough so that the baby can breathe easily, but can't really move around.

This amount of pressure should be comfortable for you. If you find that you are getting tired arms or sore hands, possibly you are using too much pressure or your chair is not at the right height. If you are not relaxed, it will be hard to give perfect support to your patient.

Someone else's baby

As a member of the PD Team often says, "The biggest mistake therapists make is that they hold their patients with Parkinson's as if they were their *own* babies: cooing over them, worrying over them. You should hold a person with Parkinson's as if he were *someone else's* baby."

Comfortable force becomes imperceptible

We can even become used to unnatural forces; when we wear clothes and shoes to which we have become accustomed, we no longer notice them: they become "forceless." Within a few moments of putting on a comfy pair of old shoes, we have no awareness of the shoes pressing against our feet.

When we wrap on an ace bandage over a weakened, sprained area, we quickly forget that the bandage is there: we very quickly stop perceiving the force of the bandage, but we move better because, deep inside, we know that bandaged area is being supported.

One excellent FSR practitioner that I know says that, when he sits for an hour not moving, with his hands cradling a PDer's wounded foot, he feels like a human cast. Actually, that is a very good analogy. Of course, a plaster of paris cast or a more modern plastic cast gives solid support, but it is rigid, cold and cannot conform perfectly to the changing contours of a live human. A "cast" made of human hands gives a far better level of support: it is warm and conforms more perfectly to the skin of the patient.

Practice time!

Ask permission to support whatever area you are going to hold.

Place your hands on your practice partner's forearm or leg and experiment with positioning your hands until you find a pose that is very comfortable for you.

Have your partner tell you if your hands feel too pushy, too light, or if they feel just right.

Have your partner then try the same on you.

Take turns seeing how it feels to hold someone's forearm. If you think you are comfortable with the forearm, try holding the upper arm. Try holding the partner's thigh or lower leg. Play with this. See what it feels like to hold supportively but without expectation, and how it feels to be held.

Above all, notice that, sometimes, especially as you get faster and more relaxed about putting a lot of pressure on right from the start, the partner's muscles will relax or move in the area where you are holding.

As you get more familiar with this type of holding, try pretending that your confidence level has increased to the point that, as soon as you set your hands on your practice partner, you are instantly applying just the right amount of pressure. In other words, you *don't* want to get in the habit of spending five minutes figuring out exactly how much pressure to use. Have confidence.

Practice resting your hands firmly and opposite to each other until you get to the point that you know, even before you set your hands on your partner, just how much pressure you will be wanting to use. From the moment you start to place your hands on your partner, do it confidently.

Working through clothes

As mentioned, this technique can be practiced on a partner's clothed limbs. At the very beginning, it may be easier for your *mind* to accept the fact that you can feel a partner's response if you are working with bare skin, so you might want to work on a partner's bared arm, to start.

Review

Delicate touch, heavy touch

Though I'm being blatantly redundant here, I repeat that touching, if done too lightly, is an irritant. Oppositely, when touching is done with too *much* pressure, so that it causes pain, it may even generate a pulling-away response. If there is one-sided pressure, as opposed to two-handed pressure, the subject cannot help but push back, instead of relaxing.

The type of touching used in FSR is the confident, *firm* gentleness with which a mother holds someone else's child while she's ignoring it by being mentally occupied with something else. FSR requires supportive contact that does not impose a command, but conveys confidence and assurance.

"Forceless" touch

Most often, the beginner is far too delicate, employing an irritating, "gentle" touch. The problem is that he is trying to be "forceless." Consider that the word "forceless" in the name Forceless, Spontaneous Release applies to the perception of the *patient*, not to the amount of pressure used by the practitioner. It also applies to the intention of the practitioner, inasmuch as the practitioner isn't using any directional force on the patient, but is just sitting there pressing his own hands against *each other*, and not applying force to the *patient*, per se.

The more pressure you use, to a point, the less the patient will notice it. When the patient perceives no directional, instructional force coming from your hands, and instead only perceives that he is being truly supported, his relaxations will be in response to this perceived "absence" of force.

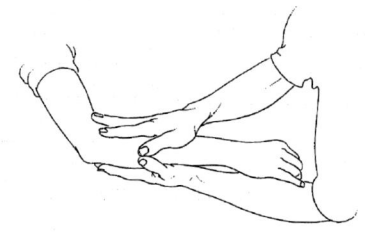

Chapter five

FSR technique: following the movement

The relaxation response: movement occurring in your partner in response to your holding

When you practice holding your practice partner's forearm, you will notice, eventually, that at the moment when you place your hands on your partner using firm support an *immediate or fairly rapid* and, sometimes, visually perceptible change occurs in the position of those muscles in your partner which are immediately under your point of contact. This comes from the immediate, localized relaxation of the patient's body part in response to your support. The change may even be *visually* perceptible to you (and your partner) because your hands, making firm contact, will perceptibly move even as your partner's forearm relaxes. While you might not be able to notice the movement in the *partner's* arm, you might easily notice that *your* hand positions almost immediately altered from the exact position in which you started.

Because of your commitment to supportive contact on your partner's skin, when his skin/underlying muscles move, your hands move along with him. If you notice that your hands are resting in a slightly different position than they were when they were very first placed on the partner's arm, then you can be assured that this is because the partner's muscles and skin have moved.

If your partner's skin moves, keep holding: follow the movement. Maintain contact, and let your hands be carried to a new position by the movement.

Lots of relaxation movement

Often, the relaxation response is small and gentle.

Sometimes, the relaxation response is a bit jerky.

Other times, the relaxation response will actually move back and forth, instead of in a simple, one-way move. Fine. Keep your hands in place until the area being held stops moving back and forth.

Now and then, the relaxation might feel as circular movement is occurring in the skin under your hands, or in the fascia that's just under the skin that's under your hands. You may feel as if one or both of your hands needs to move in a circle in order to adhere to the skin or fascia's movement.

It's actually impossible for your hand to move in complete circles while maintaining contact, so what you'll do is let your hand rotate a bit, maybe as much as forty-five degrees, following the movement. Then, when you've rotated at the wrist as many degrees as you can comfortably tolerate, quickly pull your hand off the skin and bring it back to a comfortable wrist position. Set your hand back down on the patient – and let it continue following the rotation, if any, in the patient. If the patient's fascia feels as if it's doing a lot of "unwinding," you may need to pull your rotated hand off and quickly set it back down a dozen times, or more, to keep up the sensory illusion of support without making a corkscrew out of your wrist.

The following two pictures are the first and last of a continuous photo group, with the camera mounted on a tripod. The camera started when the hands were placed on the patient. The photo group ended after two seconds, when the patient's skin stopped moving.

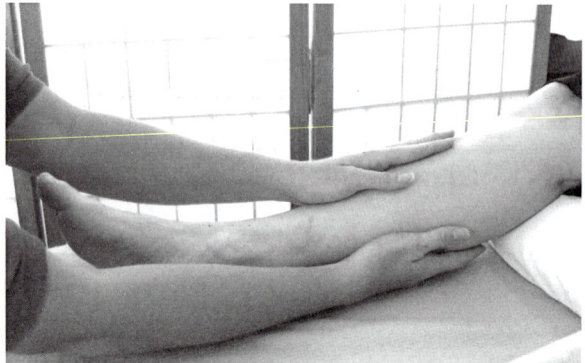

Fig. 4.3

Notice in the second photo the very slight tilt in the wrist muscles of the practitioner's upper hand. The third finger is no longer visible. In the lower hand, the index finger has rotated away from the camera, and the arm just proximal to the wrist has elongated slightly.

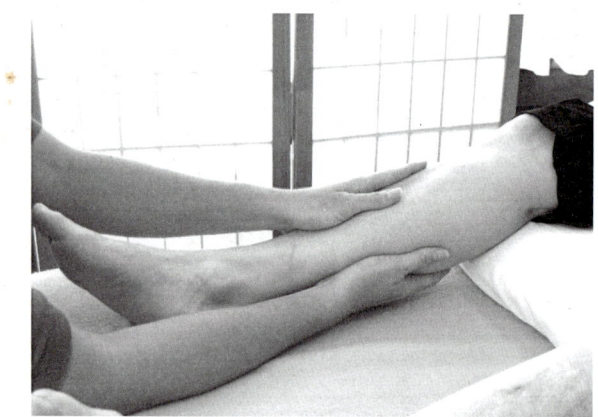

Fig. 4.4

A question

You might ask, "What if my partner is already relaxed? If so, he cannot relax in response to being held." Don't worry. If your partner is fighting gravity, he is doing work and, therefore, is not perfectly relaxed. One can safely assume that all healthy patients/partners are not in a state of perfect relaxation and *will* relax somewhat in response to being supported.

When your hands are applied to his forearm (or any body part), your hands will supplant some of the patient's inherent tension; the touched area will relax its share of internal muscular grip accordingly. This small release of muscle tension will create a movement in the skin and underlying muscles, such that the practitioner's hands will find themselves resting on the patient in a slightly different position than when they began.

This change might not be perceptible to the practice partner if he has his eyes closed. Because he felt no vector of force being applied, the partner will most likely think that nothing has happened except that he briefly felt the initial contact from your hands. If the partner sees that your hands have moved slightly in the first moment after you placed your hands on him, he will most likely assume that *you* have initiated some movement that caused your hands to move.

This may seem redundant, but here goes: even if *you* feel a significant relaxation in your practice partner so that your hands move a good quarter of an inch or more, if your partner's eyes are closed during the time of contact and subsequent movement, *he* might not detect that anything has happened at all other than the fact that you are supporting his arm. If he *does* notice that his muscles have moved, he may very well accuse *you* of having moved them. Because he did not give any conscious movement command to his muscles, it may be hard for the patient/partner to realize that his muscles moved reflexively of their own accord. It is very common for students, working on each other, to accuse the "practitioner" half of the pairing of having imposed movement on the area in question.

Sometimes enough relaxation can be inspired just through this type of *brief* holding that a significant release of tension or repositioning of displaced bone or tissue will occur. Sometimes – and this is the point – in response to this supportive touch, relaxation and awareness of the area can increase in an area that previously, due to tension, was resistant to healing.

Then again, sometimes it takes longer to get a response. In people who have dissociated from the body part in question, it can take a long, long time to get a response.

Maintain the support during movement

Holding on, keeping the hands in supportive contact even while the patient responds or moves around, is a critical part of the support. When you hold a person with supportive touch, you are rather implying that you are there for him, holding him for as long as needs be. This means that, if your patient's arm (or whatever body part) does move in response to being held, you have an unspoken "obligation" to continue to follow the movement wherever it goes, providing support until you receive a "let go" signal. Sometimes this means that a practitioner's hands may end up in a very different position than where he started. But wherever the patient goes, there you, the practitioner, must follow.

Letting go temporarily, moving to a more comfortable position

If, in response to your support, the patient's arm (or body part) moves in such a direction that you can no longer hold on comfortably or keep your balance, then, of course, you should let go and smoothly, quickly, reposition your hands in a way that will allow you to be comfortable while continuing to provide support.

The patient will not go to pieces if you let go for a quick moment.

Sometimes, if you sense that the patient's body truly does not want you to let go, but you simply must move to a more comfortable position, then rotate your arms around or move your torso in such a way as to accommodate to the new holding position without actually lifting your hands off the skin, if possible. As soon as the patient's body part stops moving and is getting settled in in the new position, you can smoothly and quickly lift your hands off and resettle them in a more comfy position.

Use your common sense with this; there is no value in having the practitioner get a crick in his neck. Picture a worried child wanting to be held tightly by a parent: the parent can move as much as he needs to get himself in a comfortable position and the child will not fall apart while the parent does so. However, once the parent gets to a position of maximum comfort and stops fidgeting, the child also settles down more deeply.

Sudden jerks

The practitioner must be prepared to hold on during those rare response movements that are large or jerky. If your hands are committed to supporting the patient and suddenly the patient's arm (or whatever) twists or bounces, you need to hang on even though you may feel, for a split second, as if you are being carried somewhere unexpected.

The warning signal

As you become more experienced with this technique, you may begin to notice that a faint electrical discharge that feels sort of like static energy moving through your own hands and even up your arms will often precede a major jerk or twist on the part of the patient. If you are in tune with this sort of thing, you can use these static discharges as a warning to brace your feet on the floor or loosen up your elbows in preparation for a sudden lurch or lunge.

An anecdote

I was holding onto a patient's upper thigh and getting no response at all. I was standing at the side of the treatment table, mentally settling in to a comfortable daydream. My hands were holding firmly on her leg, but my mind was rapidly moving to a place a thousand miles away. After several minutes, I felt a flash of static electricity in my arms, but before I could even steady myself in response, I found myself lying across her legs, my head hanging down the opposite side of the table from where I'd been standing a moment earlier. My hands were still gripping firmly on her leg, which had rotated medially so abruptly that the force of the rotation had lifted me off my feet and flung me towards the opposite side of the table.

She laughed. She had felt nothing at all in her leg even while she saw me sailing through the air, over her legs. A moment later, she sighed with relaxation and announced that she had more feeling in her leg.

This *extreme* tossing around has only happened to me once. But many times a patient's head, arm, leg, or foot has shaken me like a terrier shaking a rat.

You never can know just what's going to happen. So tell your hands to hang on, and tell your mind to relax and mind its own business.

This simple holding and the almost immediate response (in uninjured areas) that you can notice by movement occurring under your hands are the basic events of FSR. Practice it on someone else. It is very hard to practice it on yourself.

The patient's sense of what's happening

Sometimes, but not always, the partner will say, "My muscle movement wasn't reflexive: I was *consciously* doing that. I felt that I had a choice as to whether to move, or not."

This description of the inner conflict, or choice, is perfectly correct. The body might have been somewhat reluctant to move, and yet wanted to move. Healthy relaxation occurs when the person allows himself to move in the manner that the area seems to "want."

Consider this: when you firmly hold a startled, panicked child until he calms down, that child does not perceive that you have done anything to him. And yet, he calms down quickly if you hold him firmly enough, with enough confidence. So you *have* done something, and you can feel him relax in your arms as a result. But he won't have *felt* that you've done anything. Not only that, the child may be aware that he *made a choice* when he relaxed: he *could* have stayed upset, but he chose to relax because of the support that he was getting.

Sometimes, when people see me, as teacher, demonstrate this technique on their partner, they want to protest that the partner's arm movement was not due to relaxation on the part of the partner. They accuse me: "You were shoving their arm around!" I have to insist that I was doing nothing of the kind.

Other students take the opposite stand: "Nothing happened in *response* to your hands, the partner just *happened* to relax a little." Well, of course. That is the whole point: the partner will relax when supportive hands are placed on his skin. This relaxation *can* be extremely fast and it may seem to the person being held as if nothing significant has actually happened.

Because the response is so unpredictable, sometimes hard to feel on the part of the partner and so startling to the new practitioner, it is possible that both the practitioner and the partner may want to insist that the *other* person must have been intentionally "moving the forearm around."

An old, forgotten injury

If your "healthy" practice partner's arm does not respond in the manners suggested above, and especially if there is no relaxation response, it is very possible that the partner has an old injury in the arm you are holding. If so, use the other arm. If the other arm also does not respond, try having the partner lie down and work on the partner's calves.

When I've taught classes in this technique, there's usually one person out of the twelve students whose body part doesn't relax as predicted. A quick intake usually uncovers a medical history of broken bone or severe injury in the area that didn't relax in response to being held.

So when choosing a practice partner, you might *not* want to work, at first, with someone with a history of many broken bones and a "high tolerance for pain."

If your partner doesn't respond, at all, to your holding, don't worry, don't assume that you are doing something wrong. The unresponsive partner may well have an old injury in the area(s) in question *and* might not even remember the old injury. But do consider working on someone else, if you don't get any responses with your first practice partner. If you can work on several people, that would be best.

Don't be shy about recruiting practice models from among your friends; most people don't mind having their arm held for a few minutes. If someone does mind, or feels uneasy about it, that person may well have some unhealed injury or history of trauma in the arm and might not even be aware of it. *Never* force yourself on someone who does *not* want to be touched.

Often the hands will solve a mystery that the mind has struggled with in vain

— Carl Gustav Jung

Chapter six

FSR technique: a diagnostic tool

FSR as a diagnostic tool

The healthy areas in normal people have an automatic, reflexive relaxation response to being firmly held. The *injured areas* of people with Parkinson's, in stark, clearly perceptible contrast, do not have a reflexive, automatic response to being supported. This allows us to use FSR as a diagnostic technique to determine where, exactly, the unhealed injury, if any, is located.

Referring to a health technique as both a diagnostic tool and a therapy is somewhat uncommon in the western medical realm. However, when applying assessment methods that indicate whether or not a person can pay attention to a given part of his body, the very process of assessment can also be an attention-garnering act. As the body brings its attention or curiosity to an area, it may also bring healing capability to the area: the assessment becomes the therapy.[1]

---

[1] Years ago, when I was studying Zero Balancing, a moderately Yin type of body stretching, the teacher kept saying "Gently move the patient's foot (or neck or whatever) in direction X or Y and then *assess* what happens." We were never told to treat anything – only "assess" the patient to see where work was needed. Over the course of two days, I got increasingly antsy with the "assessment" process. I was eager to find out what technique we would do on the areas that had been "assessed" as needing more work. It turns out, there *was no* treatment technique! The "assessment" was the whole thing.

Not until the end of the two-day workshop did it occur to me that the actual work of Zero Balancing *was* the gentle moving of the patient that was done for "assessment" purposes: the assessment process was the technique. The verb "assess" had been used, very wisely, by the originator of Zero Balancing to prevent students from thinking that the imposed movements were supposed to *do* anything to the patient. By asking practitioners to "assess" what happened when moving the patient, the practitioners very carefully tuned in with what was going on in the patient's body, but didn't try to actively do anything. The significant benefit that was observed by patients with spinal problems was "spontaneous:" it occurred on its own, while the practitioners were very gently moving the patient around, trying to make an assessment.

I realized, several years later, that a major challenge for founders of various schools of what's called "light touch" movement is writing up the instructional material. If the founders use verbs that imply any sense of *doing* on the part of the practitioner, most of the students will cheerfully misunderstand and use some, and therefore, too much, force. On the other hand, if the writer says "assess" or "apply a few grams of pressure" (a gram being less pressure than most humans can even detect. Five grams of pressure is approximately the mass imposed by the weight of a nickel that is resting on a table.), the student *might* correctly go about his work of touching in a non-forceful manner. In many forms of light-touch body work, the patient responds *because* of the lack of imposition. You might say, in these cases, that "assessment" and the therapeutic "work" are very often one and the same.

Diagnostically speaking, *if* your patient had a relaxation response in a particular area, then that area is healthy enough, for our purposes: you don't need to work any longer in that particular area. Of course, hold it until it tells you to let go. If there *were* any lurking unhealed bits of energetic blockage or twisted fascia lingering in the area, the relaxation response and the electromagnetic "let go" response will have initiated a communication with the brain reminding it that it's time to heal any unfinished business. The body might still have some healing to do, but *your* job is finished: you have brought the body's attention to the area.

If your partner had a response, you can make a mental note of the fact that this particular body location is *able* to respond, and you can move on to the next body location, a few inches away.

For diagnostic purposes, we are not necessarily looking for one particular movement or another. What we are really looking for is the ability to respond in some manner – any manner. If an area is blocked or dissociated, it will *not* be able to respond to your touch. If it cannot respond, it also cannot fully heal. So, if it cannot respond, we want to know about it, so that we can help bring that body part back into the realm of responsiveness.

Watching for movement

Practice supportive holding on your partner's forearm and notice whether or not any response occurs, and if so, how much. This may seem redundant at this point, but though the material is similar, notice that the focus has now changed. We have moved away from "How much pressure" to "Was there a relaxation response?"

So even though you have already practiced holding, try it again, but this time stay focused on whether or not your patient responds. If he does respond, make a mental note that this area is OK, and move on to another spot.

Ask your practice partner if he has a history of broken arm or other trauma in the arm. If so, this will be a good place to practice holding. There is a good chance that the injured area will *not* respond as quickly as other parts of the arm – a learning experience.

Also, if you get a Go Away signal (more on this in the next chapter), whether your practice partner has responded or not, lift your hands off the skin and move them to a new location a few inches away. See if this new location responds. If you get another Go Away signal, move to yet another location. Or, if at the new location, you have noticed a response, or a lack of response, you are done diagnosing at the new location. Lift your hands off the skin and move your hands yet again, to yet another location a few inches farther down the arm.

By practicing FSR, a practitioner learns to quickly recognize what the normal range of responses of a healthy person feel like. He will also be able to recognize the highly pathological response that he gets when he zeroes in on an injured area from which a patient has dissociated.

In a person with Parkinson's disease, in order to discover which areas of his legs and feet do *not* respond with a somewhat normal reflexive movement, FSR is first used on his legs and feet in a fairly quick manner, looking for an area that will do *any* sort of response. Very often, even if the foot and ankle are not responsive, a relaxation response *can* be felt up by the knee, or in more "stuck" cases, up above the knee, on the thigh. After finding some spot on the thigh, knee, or lower leg that *is* responsive, the practitioner then moves down the leg, a few inches at a time, until he gets to a spot that *doesn't* respond to his holding.

When the practitioner has worked his way down to an area of the foot or leg (and later on, possibly an arm, hip, shoulder, neck, or cranial bone) that does *not* respond within a few moments, or minutes, and he decides that he is done with diagnosing, for now, and wants to work on "treatment" in this particular location, he will settle in, get comfortable, and just hold the area until it responds. The response might come in minutes, or in hours, or after a few months.

Diagnostically, the practitioner can assume that this area that doesn't respond has some sort of holding pattern – it is a problem area. As one gets better at recognizing problem areas, he might even start learning to feel the difference between the rigidity of a broken bone, the rigidity of a displaced bone, and the rigidity of a severe sprain. This will take time, but can be a very rewarding assessment tool for a health professional.

However, whether the movement is large, small, quick or slow, all that matters to us, for our diagnostic purposes, is whether or not this particular body part was *capable* of accepting the holding and capable of responding in any way, shape, or form. If it was, then the diagnostic answer is "yes, this area is healthy enough for our purposes right now," and we can move on to another area of the body.

A common mistake that students make is that they assume the response will not occur for several seconds. Students ignore that first "flinching" movement, and settle in to watch for something dramatic. *But the "flinch" may well be the reflexive relaxation response that you are looking for.*

Finally, what will you feel if the partner's muscles are already perfectly relaxed? In this fairly unusual situation, even if your hands are not carried away to a new position, you may feel something, a sense of life or a brief acknowledgement of your hands, in the body part that you are touching. You might feel a fleeting attractive magnetism, followed by a "Thanks, and now go away !"

Even though these signals are not large, this moment of attraction can be palpable to the experienced FSR practitioner's hands. The skin of the partner is not particularly moving away or toward the FSR hands; it feels more as if the skin and its underlying tissues are relaxing just a tiny bit into a different, more comfortable position. This too counts as a response.

And sometimes, even if a person is already happily relaxed and you start supporting his arm, he might sigh and relax further, all through his body, in response to your support.

As an aside, several times, when I've found a *severely* immobile area, the patient has then gotten radiology work done that revealed a broken bone. Having the radiology work isn't necessary, of course. But this secondary form of diagnostics, radiology, can be helpful in showing the somewhat numbed patient that he *does*, in fact, have an injury and he will be well served by allowing someone to help him with it, so that it can start to heal. It can sometimes be hard for a new patient to accept that your diagnostics are just as accurate as radiology.[1]

Setting standards for diagnostic tools: determining what is normal

You *must* practice on healthy people before undertaking treatment of people with Parkinson's or other syndromes being caused by dissociation or emotional fear in some body part. You must become familiar with what constitutes a "healthy" response. A short vignette will demonstrate the importance of this.

"My patients don't feel like *this*!"

My weekend FSR seminars were often attended by health practitioners, mostly licensed acupuncturists, who had already started using FSR on their patients with Parkinson's.

These practitioners were self-taught in terms of FSR. They had used my earlier edition of this text as their training manual. And for the most part, *despite* my admonitions, they had never worked on healthy people – people with normal responses.

Most of them felt that they'd already treated their PD patients "enough," and wondered why they weren't seeing some recovery symptoms.

I repeat, most of these practitioners had never bothered to practice first on healthy people. Ignoring the repeated textual suggestions that these techniques should be first practiced on healthy people, these practitioners had assured themselves that the tiny, random, small electrical cellular responses, forms of static electricity, coming from their Parkinson's patients were "normal" relaxation responses. Concluding, based on this wrong, presumed evidence of "movement," that their patients' blockages must be gone, the therapists, being acupuncturists, for the most part, had "moved on" from using FSR and were using acupuncture needles (their comfort zone) or physical manipulations on people who still had blocked injuries and the backwards-running Qi that is characteristic of Parkinson's.

As an aside to any acupuncturists reading this book, inserting acupuncture needles into backwards flowing channel Qi will not correct the flow pattern. It is a famous rule of Chinese medicine that one should "Never tonify an excess condition." Blockages and backwards running energy are both forms of "excess" conditions. Using acupuncture always increases the amperage (tonifies) in the immediate vicinity of the needles. In other words, don't ever insert needles in a current that is running backwards.

Despite their patients' currents still running awry, these acupuncturists were usually trying to use needles to correct the channel flow that was still running backwards. They assumed that this was the right course because the blockage *must* be gone: it must be gone because they had felt *movements*. So they thought.

---

[1] Years before I started doing Yin Tui Na, also known as bone medicine, my daughter broke a bone in her foot. The after-hours doctor to which I took her, *not* a radiologist, glanced at her x-ray and told me it *wasn't* broken. I told him that I knew that it was broken based on Asian medicine diagnostics. In this case, I was basing my diagnosis on the sudden sensitivity in my daughter's acupoint UB 11 – the meeting point for the bones. He was unsettled enough by my confident attitude that, next morning, he showed the x-ray to an actual radiologist. The radiologist quickly pointed to the break, at the exact location that I had described. The doctor was kind enough to call me and tell me that I'd been right, and went on to say that he had always been fascinated by Asian medicine.

They thought that, with effort, they could detect subtle movement deep inside the skin. Because there were no other responses occurring, they assumed, wrongly, that these bits of static charge must be the "relaxation movement" that I'd written about.

So, during the weekend seminars, I always had the students begin by working on each other – working on relatively healthy people.

When the students who'd never bothered to work on healthy people begin working on their fellow students, they were always astonished.

I remember one exclaiming to the room, "Oh my gosh! Is this what a normal person responds like? My PD patient doesn't feel anything like this!" This same practitioner had been writing to me for months telling me about her FSR progress with her PDer. She had said that he was was responding beautifully to her touch, and yet wasn't seeing a change in his PD symptoms. When this practitioner exclaimed this way, I asked her point blank if she had ever tried these techniques on a healthy person – as suggested strongly in my previous editions of this material. She told me, "No, I assumed I didn't need to. I'm a licensed acupuncturist, and a massage therapist. I thought I knew what it felt like to touch a person."

As a massage therapist, she *did* know what it feels like, to her, to push and shove on a person. But she'd never noticed how a patient *responds* to supportive, non-invasive holding.

In fact, with most of the students at the seminars, their PD patients were *not* yet making normal responses to touch, but the students assumed that they were. They still needed lots of Yin Tui Na therapy. But the therapists didn't know what was a healthy and normal response and what wasn't.

Oppositely, when I taught a class at the local acupuncture college, a class in general Yin Tui Na, using normal FSR as the *most* Yin example of Tui Na techniques, my students quickly, within a few weeks, felt *very* confident that they knew how to supportively hold a patient so as to evoke a relaxation response.

After a few weeks, I brought in to class, as subjects, six people with Parkinson's, so that my students could learn how to do the more slo-mo version of this technique: sitting and holding and waiting for a response from a person whose body doesn't seem to respond, at first.

Within a few minutes of snuggling their hands onto the legs and/or feet of the people with Parkinson's, the students were all wearing looks of bafflement.

One raised her hand, "What is it we're supposed to be doing?"

The other students quickly chimed in. "I've forgotten what we're supposed to do!" and "I've forgotten what we're looking for!"

The utter non-responses, the deathlike stillnesses in feet of people with Parkinson's were *so* weird, so *completely* abnormal, that all of the students felt that they'd "forgotten" what it was they were supposed to be doing.

I had to reassure the students that they were doing the technique correctly – the non-response was because of the patients, *not* because of the poor technique of the students.

So. If a person has no training in FSR, he may not realize if a patient is having a somewhat "normal" response or not. Therefore, I state again: the following techniques should be practiced on several healthy people before they are used on people with an injury-induced condition such as Parkinson's. After practicing these techniques on several or dozens of healthy people, a therapist may have enough sense of the normal range of healthy response that, when he comes across a strangely unresponsive area on his patient, he will be able to suspect that there is something wrong, such as unhealed injury, or even dissociation, at that spot. He will also be able to tell when the injured area is starting to feel healthier, closer to normal, because it will begin to move in response to support.

Immobility and non-responsiveness coming from the mind, with no injury

In some cases, FSR will elicit no response, whatsoever – as *if* the patient has an unhealed injury from which he has dissociated – but there is no injury at all – just pure dissociation from the heart.

In these cases, the person may perform "normal" relaxation responses if his mindset changes. I can usually induce such a fleeting "mindset change" by telling a goofy joke or two. I tell the joke, and within less than a minute, the leg or foot becomes responsive. As soon as the patient has time to revert back to his usual mindset of stoicism or wariness, the leg may become unresponsive again – either immediately or over the next hour or so.

Or the patient may learn to relax during FSR sessions: the leg or foot in question will relax and be responsive during treatments, but tighten back up again as soon as the treatment session is over. I have one patient whose legs stay relaxed for a day and a half, following each FSR session, before tightening back up again from fear.

In other words, if the patient has a body-wide dissociative mind-set, FSR in the legs and feet might be met with rigidity and non-responsiveness even though there is *no injury-based blockage*.

If the backwards flow of channel Qi, or the rigidity, comes and goes, there is *no* physical blockage (what we would call in Traditional Chinese medicine, "Blood Stagnation," a characteristic of which is a *fixed* condition that does not come and go).

If the patient is mentally inducing a state of dissociation, a state which can cause the foot and leg *rigidity* that is characteristic of dissociation, but nevertheless has no actual *injury* in the foot or leg, there is *no* need for Yin Tui Na, even though the leg is unresponsive to holding.

There may or may not be any benefit from Yin Tui Na in these cases. If there is a benefit, it may simply be that the Yin Tui Na helps the person learn to trust – a bit. If the patient can learn to feel safe while receiving Yin Tui Na – to the point of relaxation – it may help him to realize, or admit, that he does, in fact, feel *unsafe*, most of the time.

But ultimately, the treatment that will really help *this* type of patient is changing his own mental posture. He must do that himself.

This need for do-it-yourself change of the mental attitude also applies to patients whose injuries have finally healed, as well: after a person with Parkinson's has healed from his injuries, so that his channel Qi *can* run correctly, if he is relaxed, he may well continue to dissociate from his heart. He may do this intermittently or frequently, even constantly. We refer to this condition as "partial recovery." He may be able, when feeling safe, to once again move perfectly normally, but he will have impaired movement whenever he reverts into dissociation. In this case, continued Yin Tui Na is almost never helpful. It might allow the person to feel relaxed during the Tui Na treatment, but his brain might decide that he is only able to be safe and relaxed if someone is holding him: we have seen this.

I have never seen a patient who was able to learn to stop dissociating from his heart via Yin Tui Na. However, many patients do learn to desire the Yin Tui Na to provide temporary respite from symptoms, rather than doing the much harder work of changing their overall attitude towards perceived danger.

As an aside, one *can* learn how to feel the channel Qi that flows just under the skin. This can be a very helpful diagnostic tool in treating Parkinson's disease. If the channel Qi runs backwards *all the time*, regardless of jokes and mindset change, there is probably some sort of blockage at the terminus of that channel. The blockage is creating the electrical pattern that resembles biological dissociation. Then again, if the backwards channel Qi pattern comes and goes depending on the patient's mood, there may not be any physical blockage at all – but the patient may be able to assume death-like rigidity in the legs and backwards channel Qi flow when he is anxious or fearful.

A textbook, *Tracking the Dragon,* provides a simple course in direct perception of channel Qi: a very basic, though rarely taught, easy-to-learn art of Asian medical diagnostics.[1]

By learning both FSR (a very simple, easy to learn technique), learning how to feel channel Qi (a very simple, easy to learn technique), and learning to tell jokes or anecdotes in such a way as to temporarily disarm the patient's fear-center, a health practitioner, friend, or spouse of a person with Parkinson's can have at hand all the diagnostic tools that he needs to determine whether or not the patient does have an unhealed injury from which he has dissociated, and if so, where.

Diagnostics based on some sort of response: summary

This technique can be used diagnostically in this sense: if no response occurs, there is probably subconscious tension, physical or electrical blockage, or some sort of mental protective holding pattern such as dissociation in the vicinity of where you are holding.

What is a response? Any movement. The movement may be visually imperceptible, or it might be a big jerk. It may be accompanied by clicking sounds, as bones slide back into place. Movements might seem like the follow-through to an old impact, or do back and forth wiggling, or circular movements, or a slow glide.

Oppositely, an *absence* of movement *or* a definite electromagnetic attraction between your hand and the patient's skin, an attraction that doesn't want to let go even after ten minutes, or longer, suggests that there's something either out of place, broken, or for some other reason crying for attention in the immediate area. If so, this area may benefit from a long period of holding, or several sessions of holding – sessions that may eventually lead up to one, or several, relaxation responses.

---

[1] *Tracking the Dragon*, Janice Hadlock, 2010, published by Fastpencil.com, is a textbook on advanced channel theory and diagnostics. Available at www.fastpencil.com

If you use this technique regularly, you may become very accurate in your diagnoses: able to determine the exact locations of unhealed injuries. Furthermore, you may be able to simultaneously treat them by giving them the supportive holding that they need.

Chapter seven

FSR technique: letting go

Now that you know to keep holding on to your patient no matter where or how much his skin and muscles move around or don't move around, you need to learn when to let go. The rule is: let go when the patient's skin tells you to let go.

Your patient's skin in the area where you are holding will do a micro-electric shift when your support is no longer wanted. If you keep holding when the support is no longer wanted, the patient's skin and, soon, his mind will start sending you an electrical static message that says, "let go". However, if you are not used to observing these small but definite static signals, you may want to practice the steps below.

The "Let Go of Me" signal

Ask permission to hold some body area. Hold that area. This time, after following with your hands the movement of the practice partner's skin as he relaxes, notice that there has been a tiny, momentary sensation of connectedness between your hands and the skin of the partner. This sensation can be felt even if clothing is between your hands and the partner's skin.

The sensation might be described as feeling magnetically bonded to your partner's skin. A moment later, or maybe as long as ten minutes later, you will notice that your skin ceases to feel bonded to your partner's skin: the magnetic bond seems to be broken.

In fact, your hand may detect the opposite sensation: it may seem as if your partner's skin is pushing your hand away ever so slightly. This is the signal to Let Go.

The "Let Go" sensation is similar to the sensation of trying to put two similar magnet ends together. The force that repels the north end of one magnet from the north end of another magnet is very much like the force that a person's skin exerts on the hands of someone who has been holding on for too long.

Going back to the first feeling, the feeling of being magnetically attached, this sensation of a static connection has been compared to the feeling that exists between two socks that have been tumble dried together and have become charged with static. The socks *can* be pulled apart, but the pulling will require a small amount of force: there is a perceptible attraction between the two socks.

A similar attraction may be palpable between your hands and the skin (even through clothing) of the partner. This feeling of electromagnetic attraction occurs when the patient or practice partner's skin or muscles *want* you to continue holding.

This feeling of mutual attraction may occur before, during, and/or after the relaxation response.

Do not let go of your partner as long as you can feel that static, or magnetic pull, that seems to be keeping your hands attached to your partner.

If you try to remove your hand before that static Qi has dispersed, it will feel as if you must use a bit of force, as if you are wrenching your hand up off of the partner. It will feel somehow wrong.

If you wait until the static has dispersed, your hand will come up easily off of your partner. If the static disperses and the skin actually *reverses* its charge, your hand may almost feel as if it is being subtly repelled away from your partner.

If you feel as if your hand is being pushed away, then do not impose your hand a moment longer. Remove your hands. You are finished, at that location, at least for the time being.

Go away!

Sometimes, a "go away" signal is not an indication that the relaxation response is finished. Sometimes, a person's skin will issue a "go away" signal" immediately, even if there was *no* relaxation response. This behavior suggests that the partner is feeling very protective of this area. This may be an area that genuinely needs to be held, and will benefit from being held, but is not yet ready to be held. If this is the case, do not impose yourself on the area.

Move on. Choose another location a few inches away, and see if your patient's arm is more willing to have you at the new spot.

At some point, possibly after you've held the new spot in a non-intrusive manner for awhile, the partner's body may allow you to return to areas that previously didn't want you.

Of course, if the patient begins whimpering or trying to distract you as you prepare to hold some part of his body, don't impose yourself. Try some other area first, and slowly win the confidence of the patient.

Electric resistance to being touched

Sometimes, a person with Parkinson's will have such strong resistance to being touched, particularly in the vicinity of an injured area, that when you first begin working with him, you cannot actually rest your hands on him for the first few minutes of the treatment. Sometimes this palpable resistance to being touched can last for an hour, or may be evident at every session for many weeks.

When I have a patient with this level of fear around being touched, I might do one of several things. I might place my hands on an area very far from the injured and resistant area. For example, if the channel Qi is blocked in his legs and it seems that the blockage is down in his feet, I might hold his upper arm.

Or I might suspend my hands in the air space several inches immediately away from his injured body part. I support my hands with the muscles of my arms and shoulders, as if my hands were resting, nonchalantly, up against the electric field of his injured area that is emitting the "go away!" signal. Usually within a few minutes or a few weeks, the area is less afraid and allows me to set my hands down on the skin.

Taking too long to say "Let go"

Sometimes it will seem a bit awkward at first if you are working on a patient and a full minute goes by before you get the signal to let go. This awkwardness may be coming from completely unrelated social conventions that tell us not to shake someone's hand for too long, or not to hug a person for too long.

Please, if your skin feels as if it is adhering to the partner's body, don't worry about the social conventions for holding for too long. If the patient's body wants continued contact, go ahead and give it.

The hug that lasts too long: an example

Oppositely, when you give a social hug that lasts too long, you can (if you are sensitive to these things) feel the electrostatic repulsion force coming from that person – even if you are both wearing heavy suits. Hopefully, most of us who are planning to do this type of work already know, via our intuition, exactly how long to keep hugging someone and when to let go. Is there anyone among us who has not experienced an uncomfortable feeling when he has been hugged for a bit too long? Oppositely, haven't we all wanted, at some point in a harried or stressful day, to just be held tightly for an indefinite period – until we feel that we've had a chance to collect ourselves?

When holding small children, it is always obvious when they want to be held steadily and snugly. They snuggle in and almost burrow into your chest. And yet, the moment that they've decided that they don't need a hug anymore, they are impossible to restrain; they squirm and fidget, making it obvious that the time for holding is over. Period.

No one should need to be taught how to recognize when someone needs a hug, or when someone wants the hug to end. However, in our untouching culture, when it comes to therapeutic touch, we actually have to study and practice in order to be able to perform these basic, human functions correctly.[1]

So start practicing holding and supporting a partner's arm, leg, foot, neck, or whatever wants holding. Note carefully if there is a quick, fleeting relaxation response to the touch, and also note when the static in the skin stops pulling you in like a magnet and starts pushing you away.

Children are very quick at learning this technique. Adults sometimes take more time. Still, only a few hours of practice should be enough to get you ready to start practicing on a person with Parkinson's.

Working through clothing

Electromagnetic fields are not significantly inhibited by thin clothing, any more than a refrigerator magnet is significantly diminished by a thin piece of paper between the magnet and the door of the fridge.

---

[1] Some people *do* have trouble recognizing these signals. I have noticed that people taking certain drugs, notably antidepressants, anti-anxiety drugs, and dopamine-enhancing anti-Parkinson's drugs, are sometimes not able to ascertain when they are receiving a "go away" signal. And some people just seem to be insensitive to the signals from others, but it may be that this is learned behavior, and not a physiological lack.

The force of these fields *does* decrease over distance, whether or not there is clothing in the way. Therefore, thin clothing, which does not make a huge difference in the *distance* between your hands and the skin of your patient, will not diminish the signals being sent by the patient, but very *thick* clothing such as heavy parkas *can* diminish the sensations simply because it increases the *distance* between your hand and your partner's skin.

Relaxing all over

As you get more accustomed to paying attention to what is happening to your own hands, you may notice a feeling of relaxation in your hands, or even in your arms or torso, which occurs at the same instant that the static cling feeling goes away. As you become more comfortable doing this work, you may even begin to notice that your own body perceptibly relaxes at the same time as the partner's skin says "Let go".

Sometimes it can feel as if you had been unintentionally holding your breath, and at the moment when the partner relaxes, you find yourself exhaling, or relaxing your abdomen.

Review

When should you *not* let go? Do *not* let go as long as the feeling of electric attraction is ongoing. Do *not* let go if you feel as if your hands are being pulled in to the practice partner's skin. Do *not* let go if, when you try to remove your hands, you feel as if you have to use any force whatsoever to extricate your hands.

When *should* you let go? *Do* let go if the static or feeling of attraction has dispersed and you feel that you are no longer electrically attached to your partner's skin. *Do* let go if you feel an electric sense like that of two positive ends of a magnet being pushed at each other, repulsing each other, between your hands and your partner. *Do* let go if you feel uneasy in any way. Such a feeling of uneasiness may be coming from some energetic turmoil that has been stirred up in your patient, and, if you don't want to be a party to it, that's perfectly reasonable.

Of course, *do* let go if your partner verbally asks you to do so.

Again, in the beginning, you should not try to learn this awareness of when to let go by first working on a person with Parkinson's. The skin of a person with Parkinson's may not emit a Let Go signal for months. It may not do anything for a long, long time. The skin of a person with Parkinson's is the wrong place to learn sensitivity to shifts in electrical signals.

The absence of signals in the skin of a person with Parkinson's is closely related to the absence of signals in a mouse whose skin has been perforated by a cat: a mouse who has slipped into a state of dissociation. The absence of electrical signal in the skin of the mouse contributes to the cat quickly developing a disinterest in the seemingly lifeless mouse.

Do not look for these signals in your Parkinson's patient when you are first getting used to supportive holding and looking for signals regarding holding or letting go. You must learn to recognize these feelings on a healthy person.

It is *possible* that your Parkinson's patient will send these signals but then again, maybe he won't. At some point he may *begin* sending these electrical signals. That will be good.

But, in the beginning, learn to recognize the basic human "Hold Me" attraction force or the "Let Go" repulsion force while working on healthy people.

There are many cues that tell you whether to stay attached or to let go: the static sensation, the attractive (holding) force, the repellent (letting go) force, the partner's relaxation, and even a feeling of relaxation somewhere deep within your own body. These are all signals telling you to either hang on or let go. You may notice one or several of them. When you feel anything that is telling you to let go, let go.

You are ready to Practice FSR

You now know the basic technique of FSR. It consists of:

1. Holding: first, ask permission. Then, hold supportively: in such a way that your hand's force is met with an opposing force by the opposite hand or by some other part of your hand

2. Follow: hold snugly enough to the person's skin with your hands so that if the skin or underlying tissues move, your hands continue to give steady support.

3. Diagnose: If you get a response, even a flicker at the first moment, fine. Move on. If the person's body does *not* respond to your holding, settle in for a long holding session at that location, or make a note of the location of the unresponsive area so that you can return to it later.

4. Let go: when the patient verbally or electromagnetically tells you to let go, do so.

Get out there and practice

There is not very much about these techniques that can be taught in words. The techniques are very simple. The trick to mastering these techniques does not lie in intellectual understanding. The best way to become proficient is to jump right in and practice these biologically simple techniques. It is the practice, not the intellectual understanding, that will make you skilled.

So many students have told me, "I'm not sure what I'm feeling." The solution? Stop thinking about what you're feeling. Thinking and feeling don't go together.

Practice, practice, practice. At some point, you'll realize that your hands know what they are feeling, and convey any pertinent information to your brain, without your brain ever getting actively involved.

Practice will teach you more than any mere words can ever instruct you on this subject. Even a few hours of practice, on maybe half a dozen people, might be enough to teach you what a normal response is, and how to know when to let go, and maybe even with this small amount of practice, you'll be able to notice, through your hand's instincts, when something is "not right."

Chapter eight

Advanced FSR techniques

Holding combined with a bit of a nudge

If the person's body does not respond immediately to correct, supportive contact, it is possible that, instead of stony dissociation, only some mild tension is stubbornly residing therein. Very often, in these cases, the area under contact will not budge until some gentle suggestion disrupts the tension pattern. The area, even if it doesn't move *instantly*, *might* move and respond if it is given a little bit of a nudge.

Sometimes, a slight nudge of movement from the practitioner's hands is all that is required for the body part in question to wake up to the fact that it is being supported. Once it is awake, the recalcitrant body part may respond nicely.

Once it does move, it may be loosened up enough that, a moment or two later, it will respond to a reapplication of the simple holding technique of FSR in the normal, reflexive relaxation manner of healthy tissue.

Even without the presence of dissociation or an unhealed injury, a patient may have some little bit of hesitancy or tension, some snag in a certain area that prevents relaxation of that area. If a patient's body does not seem to respond in any way to being supported, a gentle, almost imperceptible nudge, even an *imagined* nudge of the hands may be enough to suggest to the patient that he let go of the snag. If so, you will perceive a slight movement in response to the nudge.

Then, after the initial hesitancy is gone, the patient may respond further or, in future, he will respond normally to the basic holding technique.

Diagnostically, if this spot is able to be responsive following a small nudge of the hands, this spot was *not* what you would call a "problem area". Diagnostically, the area *was* able to respond. As a practitioner, you are hunting for areas that do not respond to holding *or* to a gentle nudge. As soon as an area responds, the practitioner can move along – or linger, as one sees fit.

A bit of a nudge

What is meant by a bit of a nudge or, you might say, a tiny nudge?

The tiny movement is not really a push, it is more like a tiny bounce, or pulsing motion in which the practitioner's hands move momentarily closer together and then rebound back apart again.

Let's say that you, the practitioner, find yourself supporting your partner's forearm with your hands opposite each other. You may employ a little bit of force to bring your hands closer together ever-so-slightly. Then, *immediately* let the hands rebound back to the original position.

Note that I never use the words "push or shove on the *patient* with your hands." Instead, my language is that the hands of the practitioner come closer to each other and then bounce back apart to their starting position. The practitioner is focusing on his own hands, *not* on what is happening to the patient.

If this tiny bit of a nudge is small enough, the patient will not even perceive the force of the nudge. The nudge will not be felt because both of your hands are opposite each other, taking up the nudge pressure from each other. Since the patient is supported, he doesn't need to do any work to resist the change in pressure. Therefore, he won't really notice what you are doing.

Very often, if a slight tension in the patient is preventing the normal type of relaxation response that most people have to supportive holding, this tiny, very quick, invisible-to-the-naked-eye nudging movement will dislodge the tension. Once the tension is dislodged, the area being held may well move a bit in one direction or another. Then, the area may take advantage of the support being provided to relax to a yet more comfortable position. When this occurs, when the area starts to move, the practitioner's hands must follow the movement, continuing to provide support, as described in the section on holding on, until such time as it is appropriate to let go.

If nothing happens: *imagine* the nudge

Sometime, when the area is stubborn and doesn't even flinch or move in response to a subtle, quick nudge, you need to become *more* subtle. In such cases, *imagining* that you are pulsing your hands together for a fleeting moment might elicit a response.

Bear in mind that you are *not* imagining that the *patient* is going to move. This would be an imposition on the patient. As always, this technique allows the patient to do whatever he wants. You will imagine only that *your* hands are moving closer together, just a tad, and than rebounding to their original position.

This extremely subtle type of "movement" (imaginary) is very often the most effective type of stimulation for stubborn tensions. Very often, *imagining* that you are moving your hands as if giving a tiny nudge is the best way to wake up an area in your partner that is stubbornly stuck.

If nothing happens: change hand positions

If there is no response to the little pulsing movement, move the hands a little bit. Maybe move them a little more anteriorly/posteriorly (fore and aft), or maybe a little bit laterally/medially (side to side).

If nothing happens: try something else

You can try a few other moves with your hands if there is no response even after you try doing a gentle, two-handed nudge or an imaginary nudge. You can try shifting your hands a bit: maybe they will settle into a position that is even more comfortable, and which therefore conveys a more supportive feeling.

If nothing you do elicits a response, you can try again, using a slightly more *forceful* nudge. Every once in a while, a genuine physical push can be needed to get a response and relaxation from the person's rigid body part. Usually, if this is the case, you will know it because something in your hands "tells you" that a slight increase in physical force is necessary. In general, using more force is a technique of last resort, but once in a while, you might feel the need to do so. Don't be overtly pushy, of course. Simply bring your hands together a tiny bit more crisply than usual, using a tiny bit more force, and let them bounce back again to their normal holding position.

If this extra force doesn't do any good, it's usually best to go back to simple holding for a few more minutes to see if any sort of response will occur. If, after a bit of pulsing movements with your hands, both small and slightly forceful, nothing happens, then you can conclude that you've found a "stuck place".

Or, very possibly, after the *surrounding* areas have relaxed, the stubborn area will be able to respond.

If the stubborn bit simply does not respond no matter what, but instead sits impassively, as if it isn't really quite alive, it is very likely that an injury, subconscious tension, tissue displacement or mental dissociation has happened in this area. If this is the case, and you are still just doing diagnostic assessment, you will want to make a written or mental note of the area, and then move on.

If you have already assessed the whole area and you are returning to those areas that didn't seem to respond, then make yourself comfortable and settle down to holding this unresponsive area for a long, long time.

Advanced techniques for Parkinson's patients

When working on a Parkinson's patient, it is *very* likely that you will find unresponsive areas in the ankle and mid-foot. You might also find unresponsive areas in the knee, hip, shoulder, neck, and other areas, depending on the injury history of your patient.

Working with a person with Parkinson's can be a bit more challenging than working with a non-PD patient, because the areas that are unresponsive can cover such a large part of the body.

For example, if the PD patient dissociated from his foot when he was a child, the non-responsive area may have slowly and surreptitiously expanded to include his ankle, lower leg, knee, and even upper leg. By the time you start working on the patient, his entire leg may feel somewhat dead, wooden, and unresponsive. But you don't really want to be holding the upper leg for an hour a week, for a year, when the real problem is in the foot.

So you will want to feel over the entire unresponsive area to find that spot that feels the *most* rigid.

I usually start up by the knee – assuming that there are signs of responsiveness in the knee area. After holding the knee for a bit, until it responds, I'll place my hands a few inches below the knee, and wait for a response. If there is a response, I'll move my hands even lower down the leg, and keep going until I get to a rigid place.

If, on the other hand, the place just below the knee shows no signs of response, I may choose to stay there for five or ten minutes, just to see what happens, and to give the body a chance to get used to the idea of being held in my hands. Sometimes, after ten minutes or so, the leg area being held will respond in some manner and I will continue working my way down the leg. Other times, it will not respond at all.

If this is the case, I will give a gentle nudge, a gentler nudge, an imaginary nudge, and maybe a slightly stronger nudge. If there has been no response, I might still continue a few inches down the leg again, slowly making my way towards the spot that is more *probably* the source of the original problem: the ankle and/or foot.

With people with Parkinson's, I often find that imagining movement in my hands is just as likely, or even more likely, to elicit a response than actual movement of my hands. Then again, every patient is different.

When I finally arrive at what is most likely the real source of the problem – the actual location of injury, the original point of impact, the area feels truly different – it just feels *wrong*. You can only know what feels wrong, of course, if you have spent some time learning what feels *right*.

One way in which the location might feel wrong is that bones are obviously displaced – sticking out from the usual line of the foot, or the whole foot may be jutting to one side or the other due to a displacement in the ankle. These visually obvious displacements can be helpful. But after you've done this work for a while, the non-visible, *feel*-able vibrations given off by a frozen body part are your best diagnostic cues.

Once I get to the place where the actual injury is probably lurking, I settle in and get comfortable. Usually, my approach is to start with just holding, for a long period of time – maybe ten minutes, maybe fifty minutes. If there has been no response after about ten minutes, I might make very small moves with my hands. If there is no response, my hand movements get smaller still. Always, my goal is to be utterly imperceptible to the patient. If still no response, I might make an even tinier movement. If still nothing, I will try to keep my hands stationary and *imagine* that I am making a tiny movement. If this doesn't work, I will imagine that I am making an even tinier movement. If, after all this, there has been no response, I go back to just plain holding for another ten minutes or half hour or fifty minutes – whatever seems right at the time.

Sometimes, the patient's body can produce a Go Away signal even though nothing "positive" has happened. When this occurs, let go, and hold on somewhere else, nearby. This is not a bad thing – it shows that the patient *did* have some awareness of your hands, even if it was only a resentful one.

Other times, it may seem as if the patient's injured foot or ankle is pulling your hands deeper into his skin, as if he desperately wants even more support than you are giving. This, too, is a response, and therefore a good thing. If you get this powerful feeling that your hands are being "sucked in" to the patient's skin, then stay where you are and let your hands stick like glue until the feeling shifts or the session comes to a close.

Then again, if the patient's foot has the injury and the upper leg or knee is pulling you in, for support, don't necessarily spend all your time on that upper leg or knee. Be sure to spend more of your time on the root of the problem – usually the ankle and/or foot. When the foot finally does start to respond and the blockages in the foot go away, the upper leg will automatically get the energy and flexibility that it's been yearning for.

With PD patients, you do want to spend most of your time on the foot and/or ankle, even though other areas are calling to you. In the end, it is *usually*, though not always, the foot/ankle problem that is causing the upper leg and knee problems.

This is not always the case. I had one patient whose foot and ankle problems were pretty much resolved, after about two years of once-a-week, one-hour treatments. However, she still had rigidity in her leg and hip, so I started focusing on these areas. After a year of holding her unresponsive leg, accompanied by doses of homeopathic remedies for injury (primarily arnica), *excruciating* pain erupted in her upper leg. A massive, blackish bruise, of the type you might expect from a broken femur, appeared on her leg, and slowly dissipated over several weeks. She could not bear weight on that leg during this time. Slowly, the area healed. After that, the entire leg responded normally to FSR. Following that, I had to start work on holding her unhealed neck injury. And after that, I moved on to the cranial injury she'd incurred when a large rock was dropped on her head, when she was six years old. And so on. She usually noticed improvements in localized movement after an area had "cleared up," but her tremor – and her fear – continued.

But many people with PD have only the foot and/or ankle injury holding the PD symptoms in place – together with any dissociation from the heart that might be in place, as well. Then again, you just never know exactly what is lurking inside the body of a person who has led an active life and who has been dissociating from injuries.

Getting back to the amount of nudging that you might do: if there has been no response to any of the nudgings, don't try them again right away. It may require weeks, even months, of holding treatments before the PDer becomes responsive. Too much nudging and messing around can actually cause increased defensiveness in the PDer, and increase the total amount of time needed for therapy.

Do not try to stare down your patient's unblinking foot

Don't forget: your attention is on your own hands, by the way, and not particularly focused on the patient. Don't be scrutinizing the patient too severely. A watched pot never boils and a sensitive person or silverback gorilla does not like to be stared at. You can learn to be aware of whether or not a patient has responded without conveying to the patient that his every move is being assessed. Be somewhat detached, like the sailor that shifts and sways ever so slightly in response to the movement of the ocean, even though he is not paying conscious attention to the ocean.

Chapter nine

Foot and ankle work

This chapter has some specific holding suggestions for ankle and foot. Although people with Parkinson's may have neck, shoulder, hip, arm, cranial and spinal injuries that will benefit from treatment, and *might* need to be treated in order to recover, they almost *always* have foot injuries. Not only that, if the foot injury is causing a blockage at the intermediate cuneiform bone or vicinity, it is contributing to, or in some cases solely responsible for, those backwards flowing electrical currents that are seen in idiopathic Parkinson's. Sometimes other foot and ankle injuries also contribute, and the mental/emotional dissociation from the heart may be producing backwards-flowing currents, as well. Still, in our clinics, we usually end up zeroing in on the almost-always present Unhealed Foot Injury at the intermediate cuneiform.

The following drawings of the foot bones may help you feel familiar with the "terrain" as you start to hold your patients feet. The first drawing is a top view of the foot, with each of the bones labeled. This drawing, a simplified diagram of the foot bones, is provided to familiarize you with the names of the bones and their approximate locations.

What follows are more, detailed, dimensional drawings of the foot bones viewed from seven different angles. The detailed diagrams give a better sense of how the joints actually fit together in three dimensions.

Notice the intermediate cuneiform bone

As you peruse the drawings, note in particular the size of the middle (intermediate, 2nd) cuneiform bone in all the drawings. This center-of-the foot bone is supposed to move up and down freely during every footfall, enabling the foot to be somewhat arched or flat, at any given moment. Because of its tremendous freedom of movement, this bone is the one that is most often displaced during foot injuries.

This bone is also the end of the Stomach channel, the point from which the Stomach channel bifurcates, one branch flowing down to the toes, another branch flowing over to the side of the foot. Obstructions to electrical flow in the vicinity of this bone, obstructions such as torn or displaced tissue, scar tissue, and emotional inhibitions, can cause the Stomach channel to reverse course and run backwards – up the leg.

Also, during healthy, normal biological dissociation due to life-threatening injury, it is from this point that the energy in the Stomach channel flows backwards, moving towards the head. And when a person dissociates from his heart – you guessed it – it is from this point that the Stomach channel begins running backwards.[1]

---

[1] As a physiological aside, the backwards flow of the Stomach channel during dissociation is the reason that nausea is a common side-effect of shock or body-wide anesthetic. When the Stomach channel flow is suddenly switched from the correct direction to the backwards direction, the Stomach itself stops receiving electrical support. When a person's stomach ceases to receive electrical

Observe that this intermediate cuneiform bone is quite substantial when looking down on it from the top view of the foot (fig. 9.4). It looks like a good-sized "square" bone. The view of the same bone from the underside (plantar side) of the foot (fig. 9.8) will show you that this bone so severely wedge-shaped from top to bottom that it tapers nearly to the point of disappearance by the time it gets to the underside of the foot; all that can be seen of it is a tiny sliver, tucked almost under the 1st cuneiform bone.

"Ankle bones"

As an aside, in the drawings that follow, the ankle bones are not pictured. To be perfectly accurate, the ankle bones do not exist as separate bones. The ankle bones are actually knobs at the distal ("moving away from the torso") ends of the two long bones in each of the lower legs. These knobby ends of the leg bones nestle into either side of the talus bone, as well as sticking out to the sides, forming the protrusions that we refer to as ankle "bones".

---

instruction, the person may experience a decrease in appetite. In a case of severe dissociation, shock, or anesthesia, the person may automatically eject any food that might be in the stomach.

People with Parkinson's, whose Stomach channel flow has gradually, over decades, been altered, do not necessarily have constant nausea. However, many people with PD do have diminished appetites and have trouble maintaining a healthy weight.

A. Calcaneus
B. Talus
C. Navicular
D. Cuboid
E. Medial (1st) Cuneiform
F. Intermediate (2nd) Cuneiform
G. Lateral (3rd) Cuneiform
H. 1st Metatarsal
I. 2nd Metatarsal
J. 3rd Metatarsal
K. 4th Metatarsal
L. 5th Metatarsal
M. 1st Phalange 1st toe
N. 1st Phalange 2nd toe
O. 1st Phalange 3rd toe
P. 1st Phalange 4th toe
Q. 1st Phalange 5th toe
R. 2nd Phalanges

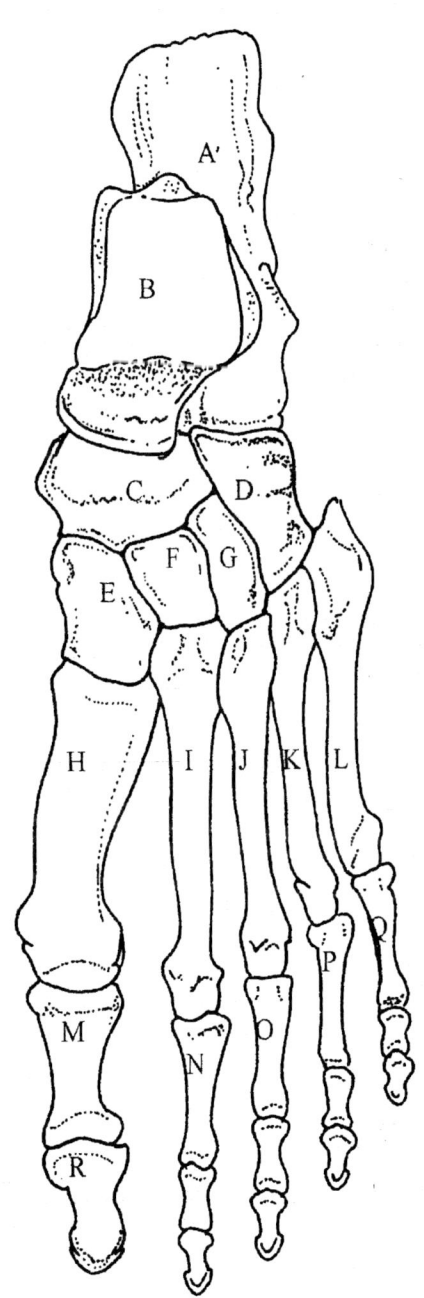

The bones of the foot
Fig. 9.1

Fig. 9.2

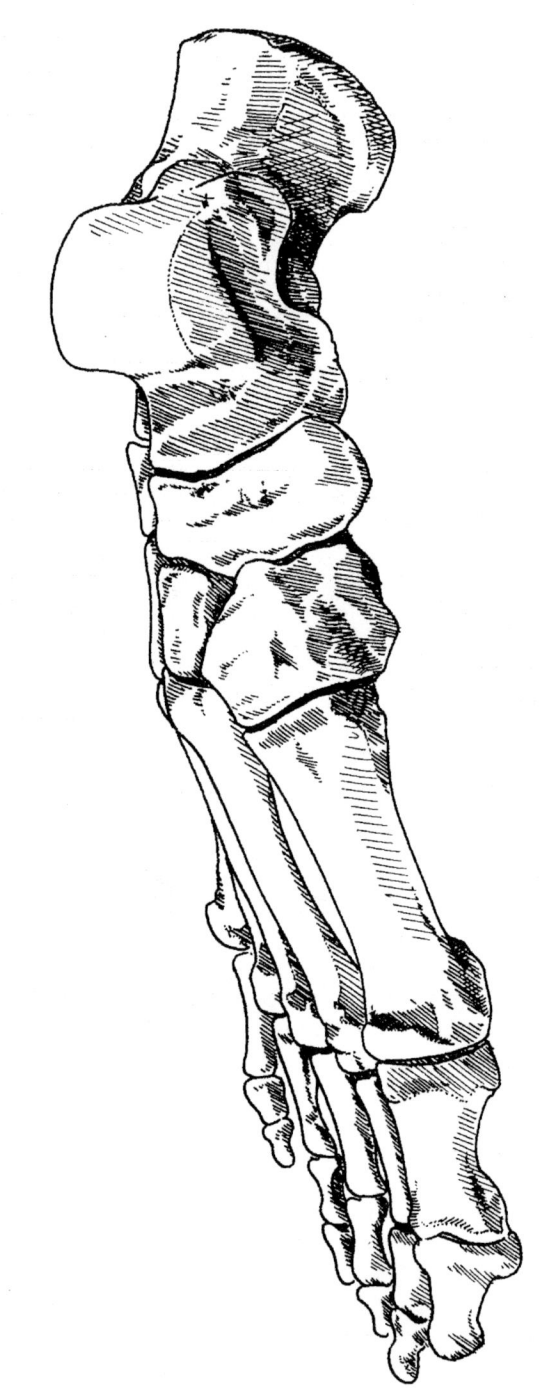

Position 1: Medial-side view of the foot

Fig. 9.3

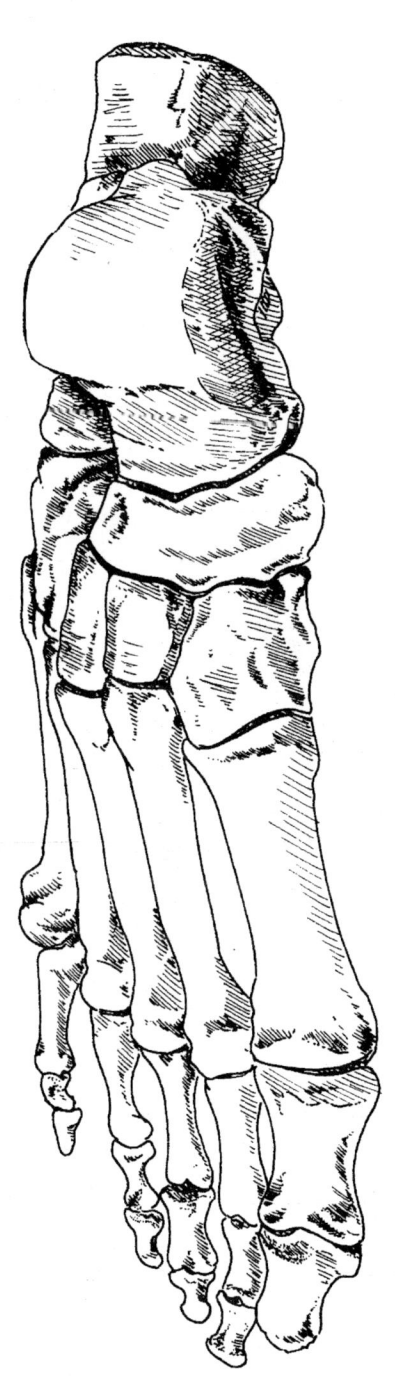

Position 2: Foot rotating slightly medially

Fig. 9.4

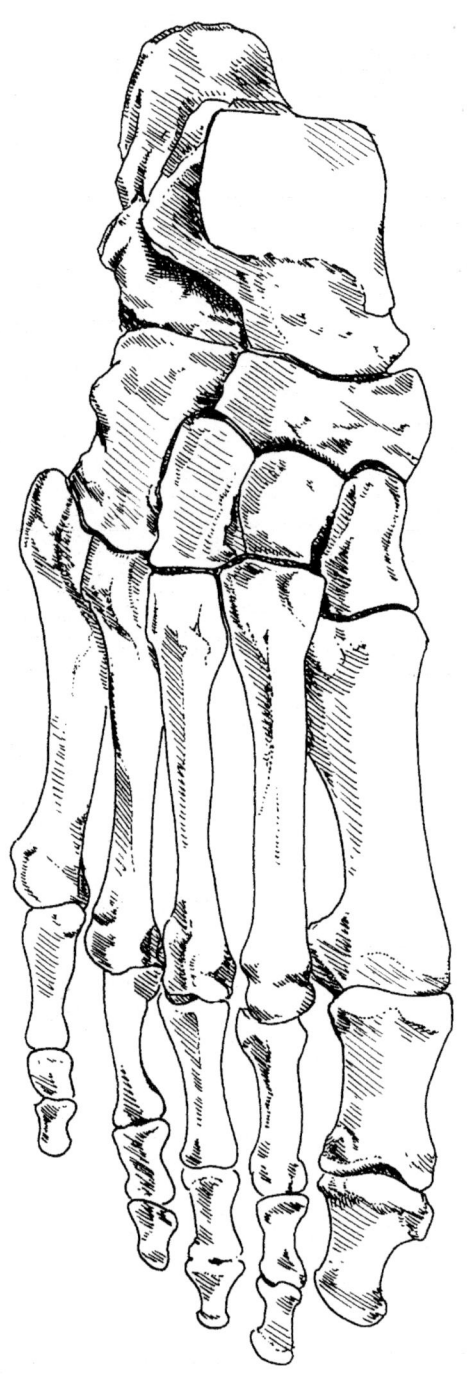

Position 3: Top view of the foot

Fig. 9.5

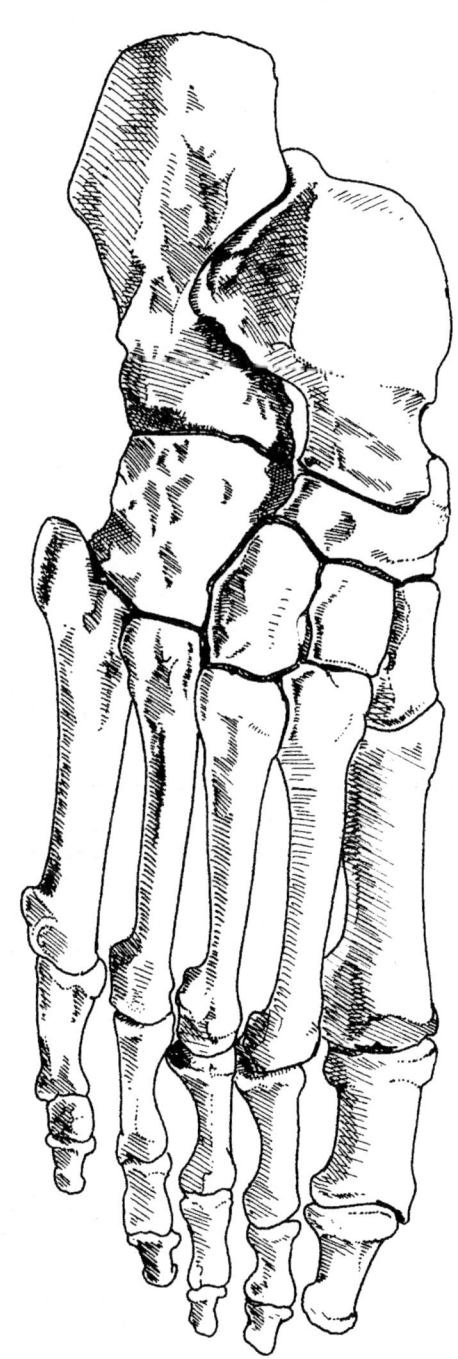

Position 4: Continuing rotation

Fig. 9.6

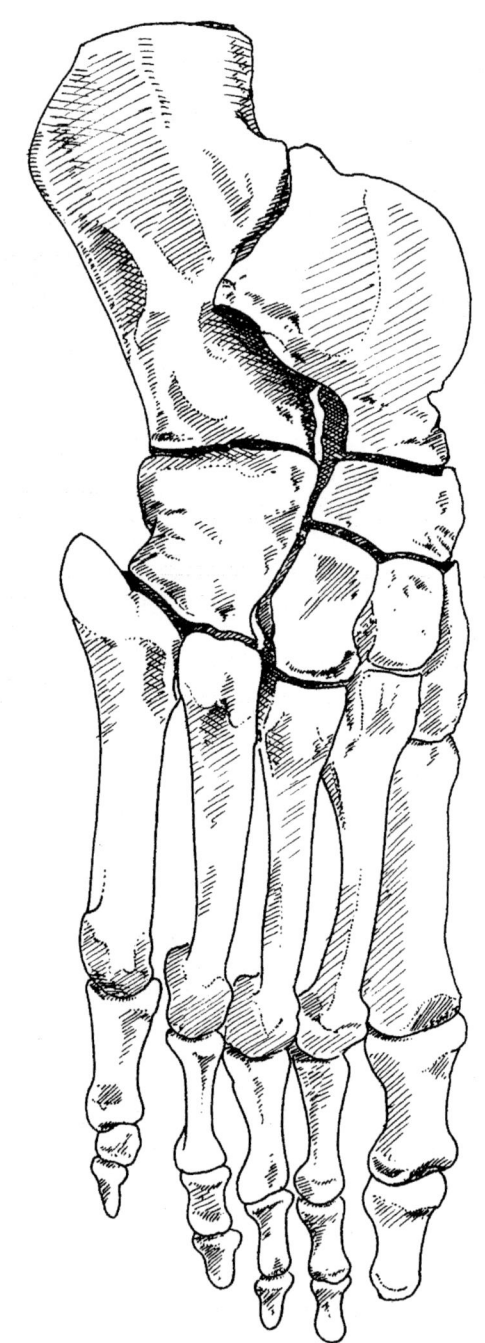

Position 5: Continuing rotation

Fig. 9.7

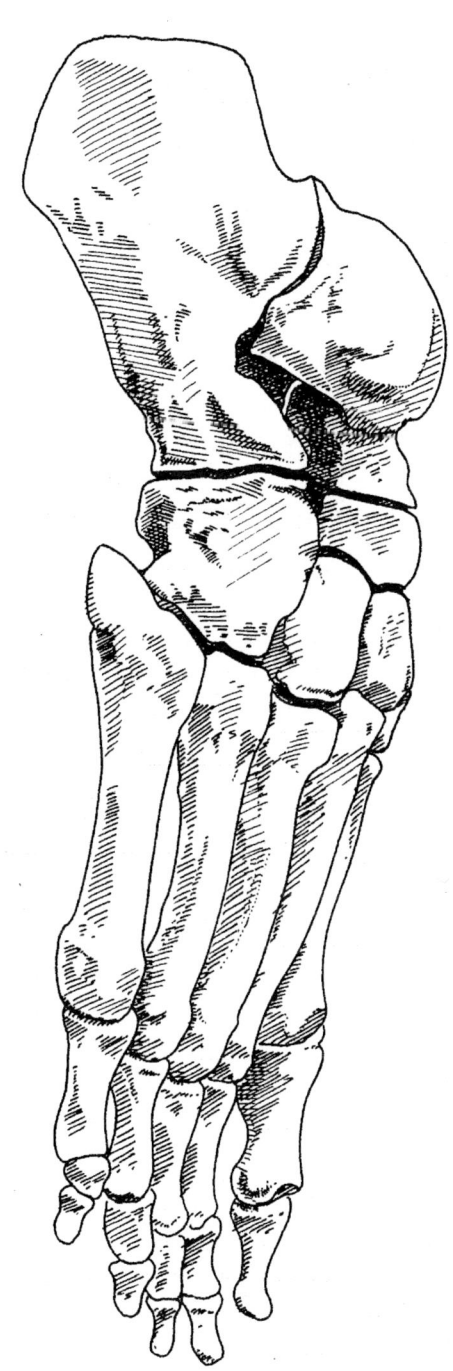

Position 6: Lateral-side view of the foot

Fig. 9.8

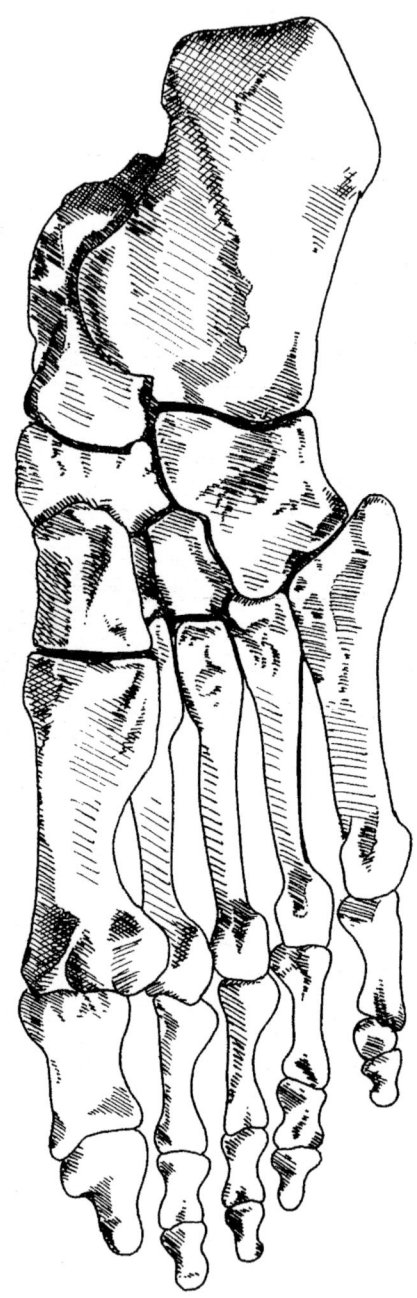

Plantar view (looking at the bottom of the foot). Note the thin sliver of the intermediate cuneiform bone, nestled in between the 1st cuneiform and the 3rd cuneiform.

Suggestions for where to place your hands on the feet

After you've quickly, or slowly, worked your way down the leg and noticed whether or not it responds, you will end up at the ankles and feet.

It was relatively easy to describe "where to put the hands" when working on the arms and legs – place one hand on any side of the arm or leg and then place your other hand opposite the first one.

But when it comes to the ankles and feet, it becomes much harder to explain exactly where the hands might want to go. Within a few hours of practicing, it may become obvious – your hands will know what to do, even if your mind does not. But in the beginning it will seem easier to you if there are a few suggestions of where to place your hands.

Then again, I am almost hesitant to describe where, exactly, to place the hands when you've moved all the way down the leg to the ankle; many students cling too rigidly to whatever I write, particularly when I describe some ankle and foot holds, even though I state over and over that the following are just suggestions. But some people are so unaccustomed to holding feet and ankles that they truly do not know where to start. This chapter provides the suggestions for places that a practitioner can hold his hands. As you become more accustomed to holding and feeling, you will soon learn where to place your hands for the best results.

The following list of possible places that you might want to put your hands also includes suggestions for directions in which you will perform your extremely gentle nudge, if any.

Again, the only reason for resting or nudging one's hands in these suggested positions is to determine whether or not the touch evokes a healthy response. You are *not* trying to forcefully move any bones, force looseness upon anything that feels tight, or force a displaced bone to its correct position.

The following suggestions will help you assess which areas might need more holding and if they need a different type of holding. If the areas do not respond to holding or nudging, they may be needing the "just sitting there, holding" variant of FSR that we use on people with Parkinson's, or with dissociation from injury.

If you want to place your hands in different places than the ones suggested, do so. The following suggestions are merely to get you started.

Ankle and foot holding/nudging positions: some suggestions

Place a hand on either side of the ankle, with the medial and lateral malleoli (ankle bones) each held snugly in a palm of your hand. If the ankle area feels responsive to your touch, good: you can move on. If not, make a note of it and move on. You may wish to return to this area later.

Next, to find out about the ankle articulations, you may want to try nudging – or thinking about nudging (usually more effective) – the ankle bones in a few different planes of movement.

Don't try to dwell on the structures of the articulations. Just notice that the ankles move or don't when you gently nudge them in various directions.

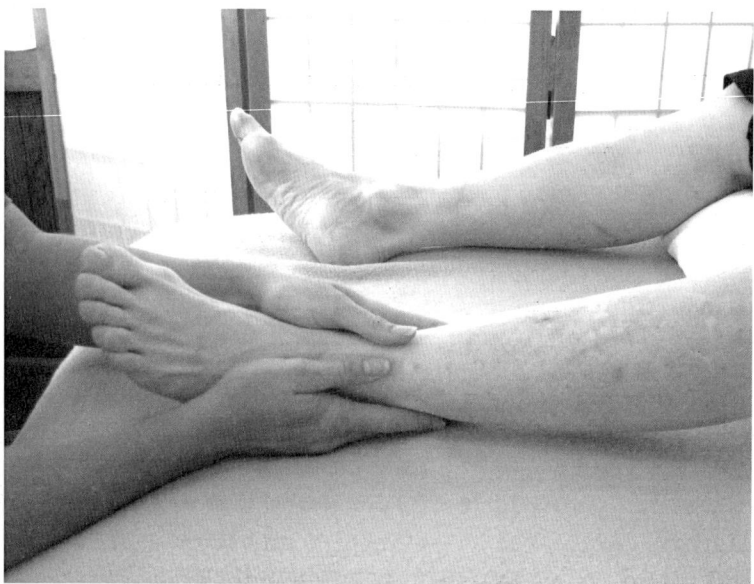

Fig. 9.9 Holding the ankles

You may wish to push your hands that are holding the ankle bones towards each other and note if the ankles respond by moving in the opposite (outward) direction. You may wish to see if the ankle bones will nestle closer to each other as a rebound move when you imagine that your hands, closely connected to the skin of the ankle bones, move slightly apart for a moment. Moving your hands apart is the opposite of nudging them together.

You may also want to try mentally moving your hand in such a way as if one of the ankle bones, for a fleeting moment, would be nudged upwards, towards the thigh, while the other one moves downward, towards the heel. See if there is any sign of a response. If not, make a note of it. If there was no response, you may want to return to this area later. If there was a response, you still might want to keep holding the ankle so see if there is a response when you think about moving your hands forwards and backwards relative to each other, and then the reverse.

The main thing you will want to do is practice doing these directional suggestions on many healthy feet so that you can ascertain just how a normal set of ankle bones moves in relation to the leg bones, the heel bone, the talus bone, and each other. Even if you don't know how all these bones should move in theory, if you hold enough feet and try mentally moving your hands over most of the areas of the feet, you will soon come to have a sense of what a foot should feet like, and how it should respond to being held.

When you've finished assessing/holding the ankles bones, you might want to move on to the heel.

84

Holding the heel bone

heel

One way to hold the heel bone is one hand under the calcaneus (heel bone), holding that round ball of the heel cupped in one hand, with the other hand supporting the Achilles tendon from behind.

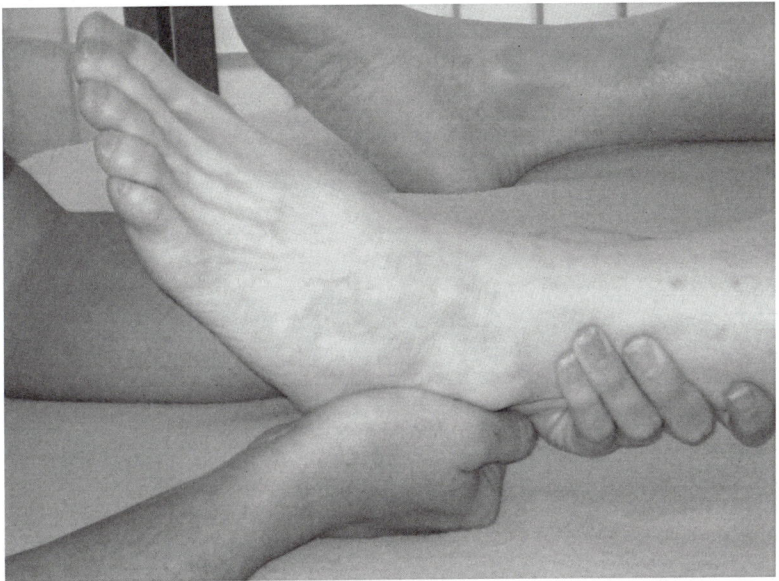

Fig. 9.10 **Holding the heel and the Achilles tendon**

Notice: are you holding a healthy, responsive ankle/tendon? If yes, then good. But if nothing seems to be moving, or this intersection of the Achilles tendon and the heel bone seems uncannily rigid, you may want to gently and quickly nudge or imagine a nudge as you bring your hands together and then let your hands rebound back into position.

In this case, your hands will be bringing the calcaneus a bit closer to the Achilles tendon. Or you might think of it as bringing the tendon closer to the calcaneus. It doesn't matter. The main thing is to notice if there's any sort of response.

As before, if a gentle nudge gets no response, wait half a minute or so and try a mere mental nudge. If still nothing happens, wait half a minute and try a slightly stronger nudge.

Also consider moving your right hand posteriorly (towards the back) while your left hand moves anteriorly (towards the front). And then try the reverse, right hand anteriorly and left hand posteriorly.

And what happens if you nudge, or mentally nudge one hand to the left and the other to the right, and then the reverse? Learn how healthy feet respond to this sort of play, and then, when you meet your Parkinson's patient's foot, you will have a sense as to whether or not all is well in this area.

If all is well in the ankle, a movement or thought that *compresses* the joining of the calcaneus and Achilles tendon, bringing them closer together, should evoke a rebounding apart in the ankle after you are done nudging. Oppositely, a nudge that suggests pulling the tendon/calcaneous junction *apart* should evoke a coming together of the two parts. In either case, the area should respond.

Eventually, in response to your holding or nudging, the heel bone/Achilles relationship may begin to feel responsive. If it does, then good. If not, make a note to yourself that this area might want some deeper work at a later date and then move on.

On the other hand, you may feel that slightly nudging (or thinking about nudging) the heel sideways to the left while thinking about moving the tendon to the right (or vice versa) one more time would be a good thing to do. Fine. Do it. Possibly by getting the heel/tendon relationship to loosen up by moving from side to side, the relationship will also loosen up in other directions as well. Do what you like, do what your intuition tells you to do, do what the patient's ankle tells you to do. Let go of the ankle if the patient's ankle tells you to let go.

Try some or all of these suggestions on healthy feet so that you can learn to understand how this tendon/heel relationship works when everything is moving nicely.

The Talus-Calcaneus relationship

Next, if you are satisfied that the heel/tendon was moving properly, or you decided that it wasn't and you made a mental note to return there later on, you might wish to place one hand on the talus bone and the other behind the corner of the calcaneous. Or you may wish to choose some other area to hold. These are just suggestions. *heel*

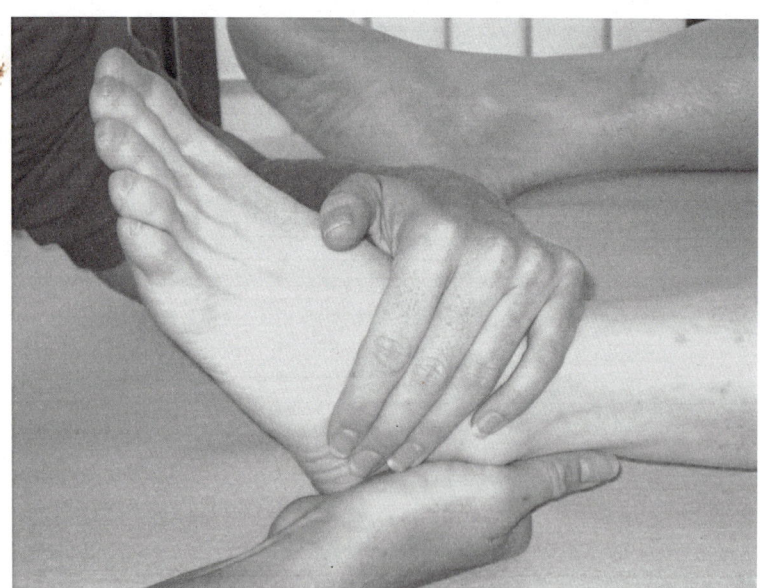

Fig. 9.11 Holding the talus and calcaneus bones
heel

Do the usual routine on these bones to assess whether or not they can move. The "usual routine" means that you will notice if the foot feels responsive when you support these bones. Then you will gently nudge these bones towards each other. Or possibly, you will gently imagine them moving apart. Or you might nudge them or imagine them moving one to the left, the other to the right. Or you might think that one is moving towards the head and the other is moving towards the toes. You can try to test these bones on any directional plane that you can imagine.

When you work on a healthy foot, by gently provoking a reflexive response in every possible direction you will be able to create a mental picture of the way that these bones can and should move, relative to each other.

An aside: foot bones make very small movements

Do bear in mind that even if these bones can move correctly, they may not move very far. They may jerk around, but they may move just a *tiny* bit, making a barely perceptible response. Of course, there is always the possibility that they will make a generous sweeping relaxation movement. But you should have no expectation, one way or the other.

Your hands, only through experience, can eventually know what it feels like to work with a responsive foot. The movements, tiny or languorous, that do occur will feel "right" to you if they are right. If you do the nudging and the imagined nudging and nothing happens, if you do the tiny pushes and pulsing and you get a sense that the bones involved are putting their backs up and saying, "No!" then you will know that this is an area that wants more work. Don't try to change its mind; just make a note that this area wants more work and go on to the next place. Or stay here and hold for a long time.

Navicular-Calcaneus relationship

Next, you may wish to place one hand on the navicular bone and the other behind the corner of the calcaneous. Again, determine whether or not this area can respond.

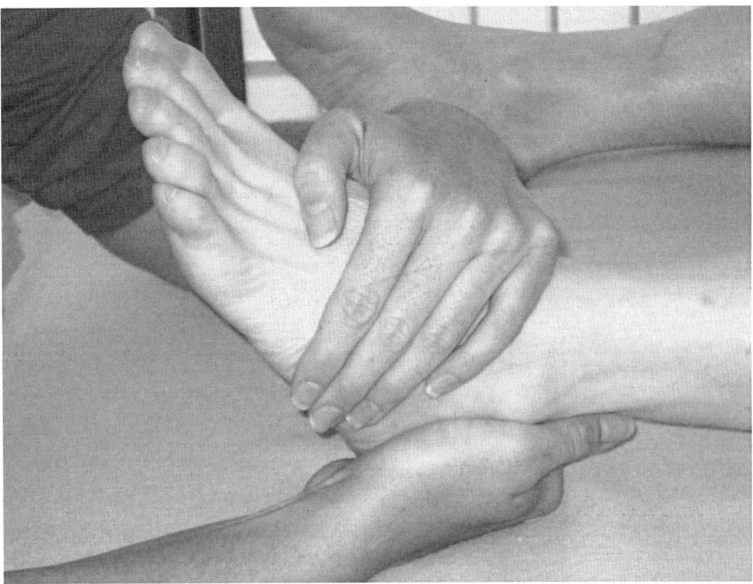

Fig. 9.12 Holding the navicular and calcaneus bones
heel

In terms of finger/hand placement while doing this, you may wish to put one hand on the navicular bone and the other on the talus. Or you may want to drape the middle finger of one hand over the navicular bone with the thumb of the same hand supporting the sole of the foot.

Or possibly, you will find that placing your thumb over the talus and the rest of the hand around the back of the ankle may feel the best for you.

If the foot doesn't relax in response to supportive holding, you may try gently pulsing your hands together in such a way that the navicular and talus bones are pressed towards each other. Or you might try thinking about your hands pulling apart from each other. Or move one of your hands that is over a bone to the left and the other to the right, or move one of them towards the front of the foot and the other towards the back.

An aside: working with less than a full hand

The curves of the foot are often so small that it is impossible to place the entire hand over some foot part. For example, when supportively holding the big toe, sometimes you can only fit a little bit of your hand around the toe, or maybe you can only fit one finger up against one side of the toe and another finger on the other side of the toe.

Likewise, because of the curve of the foot's arch, it may be impossible to place the whole palm of your hand firmly up against the bottom of the foot. In this case, instead of using your palm, you can nestle the gently curved *backside* of your hand up against the sole of the arch. In other words, the important thing here is the supportive contact, not which part of your hand or how *much* of your hand you are using to provide the support. For that matter, sometimes when I am working on a patient's foot and I sense that the patient would feel more supported if I had a third hand, I press my shoulder gently up against some part of the sole of the patient's foot while I am using both hands to support the ankle.

I am so short that, sitting on a stool at the foot of the treatment table, the table comes up to the middle of my chest. My shoulder is only a few inches higher. If the patient's foot is close enough to the edge of the treatment table, I can lean forward, causing the patient's foot to press up against my shoulder, thus using my shoulder as a third hand.

I am not saying that you need to do this. What I am trying to get across is that the patient must feel supported by human touch, and it is your job as practitioner to provide the support. A supportive pillow is not the same as a human hand. But sometimes, that "human hand" doesn't need to be the full palm of the hand, or even a hand, per se. A mere finger or a human shoulder can sometimes serve the function of a hand.

People with Parkinson's will not get the therapy they need from supportive pillows or inanimate objects. They don't need foot braces. For that matter, orthotic devices in the shoes usually do more harm than good.

People with Parkinson's, like people everywhere, do need human support. If your palm doesn't fit comfortably onto the area that you are working on, use whatever part of your hand does fit, so that you can provide support, support, support.[1]

---

[1] I treated a patient who had impaled his foot on a pitchfork. The fork entered his foot from the front, slicing in between the first and second toe and drove in deeply to the center of the foot. The injury had occurred many years earlier but the white scar was still quite visible between the toes. There was no way I could place my entire hand between his toes. Instead, I wiggled my index finger into the space between the first and second toe. My other three fingers looped around the bottom of the ball of the foot and came to rest on the medial (inside) side of the big toe. My thumb pointed towards my index finger and was somewhat wedged into the groove that runs between the toes and the sole of the foot, under the three lateral toes. My other hand was holding his ankle. I just sat like that for the full

Cuboid bone

Place the palms of one hand over the top (dorsum) and the palm of the other hand over the bottom (sole) of the cuboid bone. Look for a response.

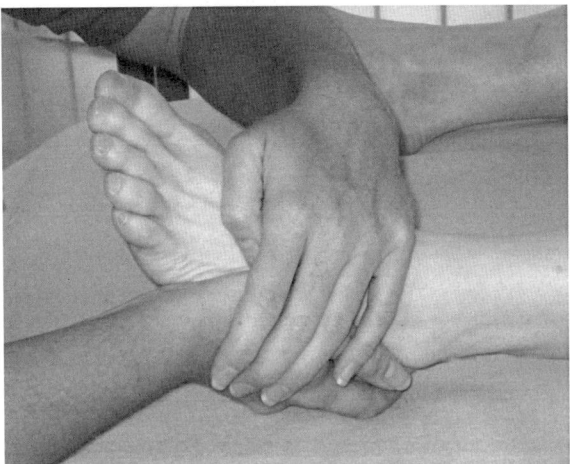

Fig. 9.13 Holding the cuboid bone

And/or place one hand on the lateral side of the cuboid bone. With the other hand, grip the navicular bone between the thumb and middle finger. If there is no response, quickly and gently compress the bones towards each other and release.

Or hold it any way you like. Be comfortable.

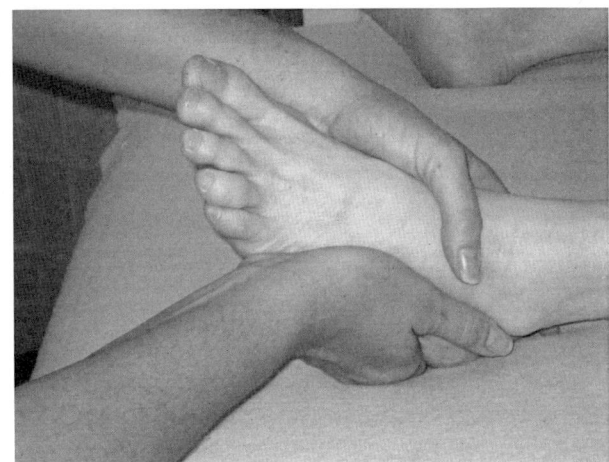

Fig. 9.14 Holding the cuboid bone

---

hour, giving very firm support to the area with the pitchfork scar. After several weeks of holding just like this, during a holding session, the entire foot relaxed, all the toes, especially the first and second, separated wide apart, and the patient reported feeling warmth and life spreading throughout his foot.

This example is provided to show that it is not always necessary to get the whole hand onto an injured spot. I was using only my index finger on the spot indicated. But the whole rest of my right hand was also providing support, and my left hand was bringing up the rear by supporting the ankle against the pressure being applied from the front end of the foot.

The cuneiforms

Place the palm of each hand on either side (sole and top of the foot) of the medial cuneiform. Compress (nudge) and release.

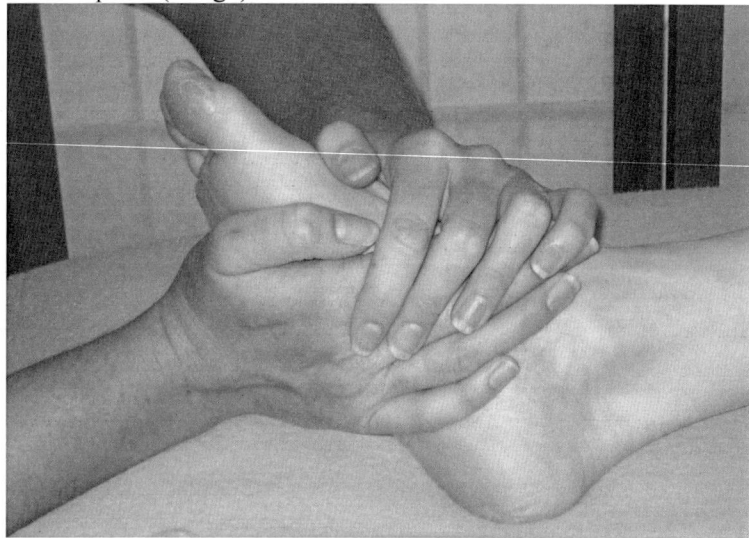

Fig. 9.15 Holding the medial cuneiform bone

Place the palms of the hands on either side of the intermediate cuneiform bone. Compress and release.

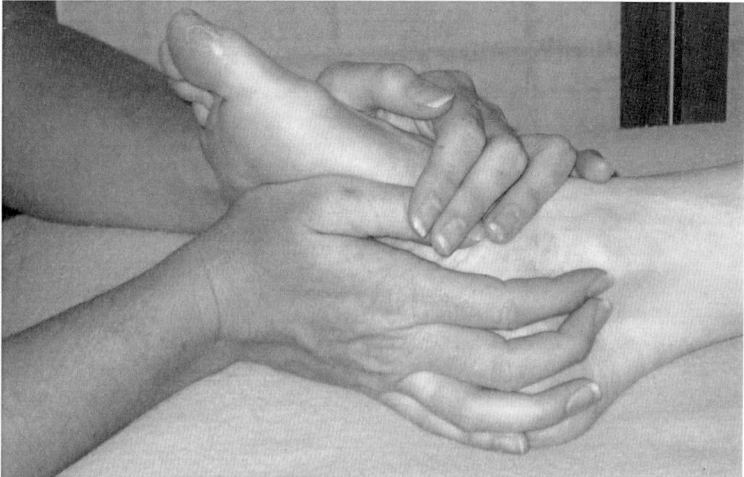

Fig. 9.16 Holding the intermediate cuneiform bone

Somewhere between your first and your hundredth treatment on a given person with Parkinson's, this bone may shudder or jerk or possibly even whip around. Until then, just do all the above supportive holdings and note whether or not the area is capable of responding.

The first time your work on a PD patient, it probably won't be. As always, make a mental note of this and plan on simply holding in this area for a long time.

On the other hand, if the intermediate cuneiform bone falls back into place, the cuboid might suddenly slide back into position, as well! In that case, the next time you revisit the cuboid bone it will be setting nicely, and perfectly responsive, even though you haven't yet worked on it directly.

Lateral, also known as 3rd, cuneiform bone

Place the palms of the hands on either side of the lateral cuneiform bone: one hand on top of the foot, the other hand on the bottom (sole) of the foot. As mentioned before, if it feels stodgy or stubborn, try gently nudging your hands towards each other to see if the foot tissues between your hands will push back outward on your hands.

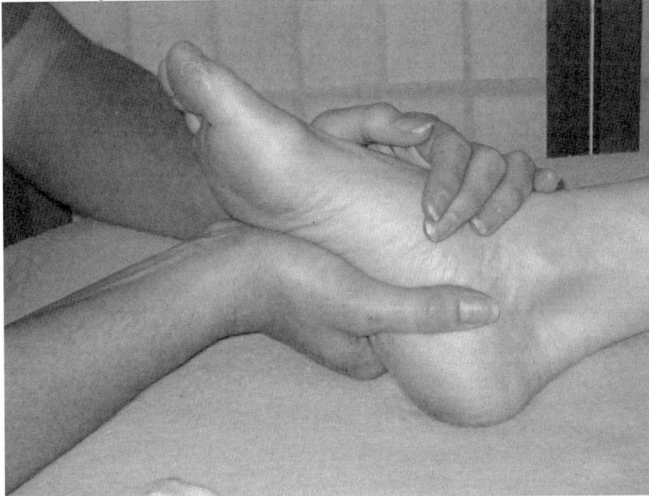

Fig. 9.17

Holding the lateral cuneiform bone

All three cuneiforms at once

Place your palm or the middle fingers of both hands over either side (top and sole) of the cuneiform bones as a group. Compress and release, (nudge) either physically or in your imagination.

Fig. 9.18 Holding all three cuneiforms at once

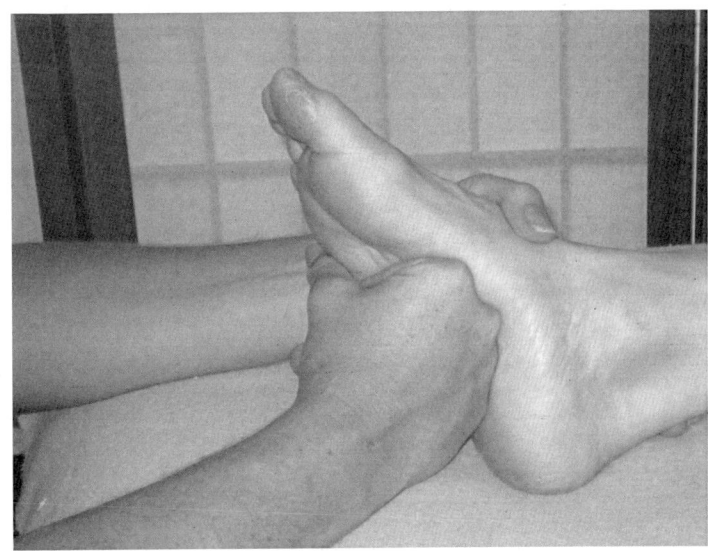

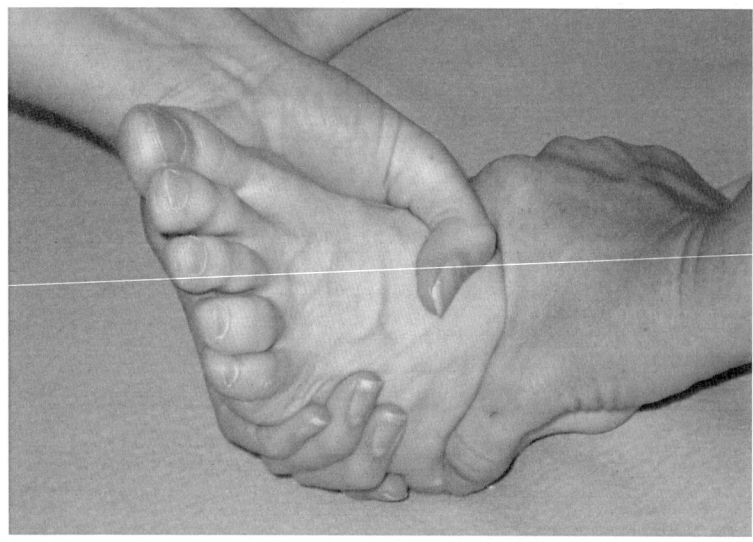

Fig. 9.19

Holding all three cuneiforms at once – a second approach

Or you might grip the cuneiform bones with one hand (thumb and middle finger over the top and sole) and grip the navicular bone with the other hand (top and sole). Nudge the cuneiform bones, as a group, towards the navicular bone and release – or towards the metacarpals and release.

Metatarsals: the long skinny bones of the feet

Place a hand on either side (top and sole) of the proximal (closer to the head, farther from the tips of the toes) end of the 1st metatarsal. Compress your hands towards each other and release. Move the hand so that the center of your palm is centered over the 2nd metatarsal and repeat. Repeat in this manner over the proximal ends of all 5 metatarsals.

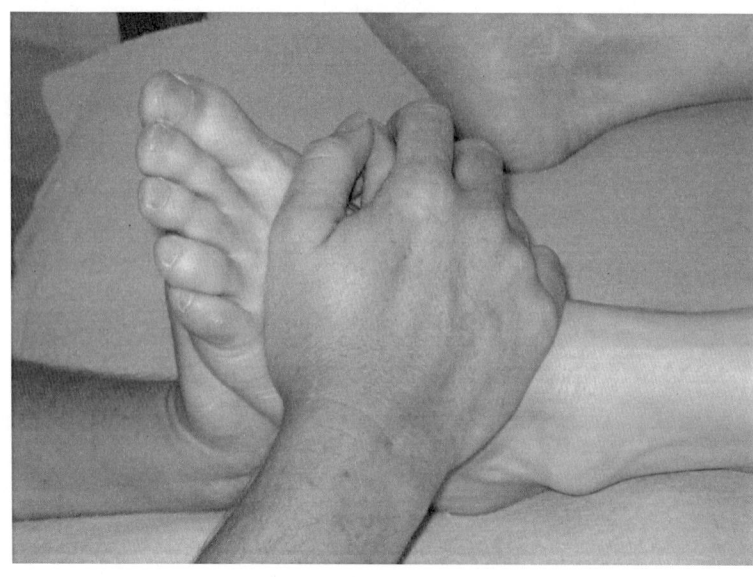

Fig. 9.20

Holding the proximal end of the 1st metatarsal

Place the palm of either hand over either side (top and sole) of the *distal* (farther from the head, closer to the tips of the toes) end of the 1ˢᵗ metatarsal. Compress and release. Repeat for all 5 metatarsals.

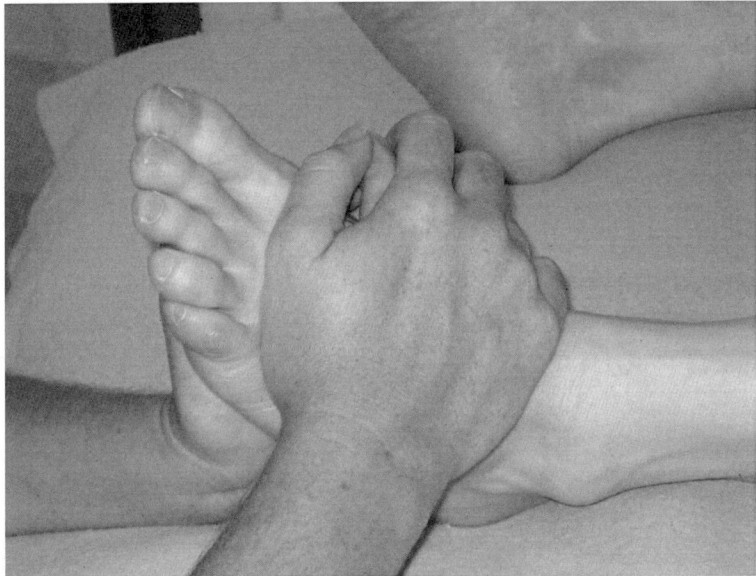

Fig. 9.21 Holding the distal end of the 3rd metatarsal

Metatarsal- cuneiform joints

Grip the cuneiforms with the thumb and middle finger over the top and sole. With the thumb on one side and index and middle finger on the other, grip the proximal end of the 1ˢᵗ metatarsal. Compress the metatarsal towards the nearest cuneiform and release. Repeat this with the other 4 metatarsals.

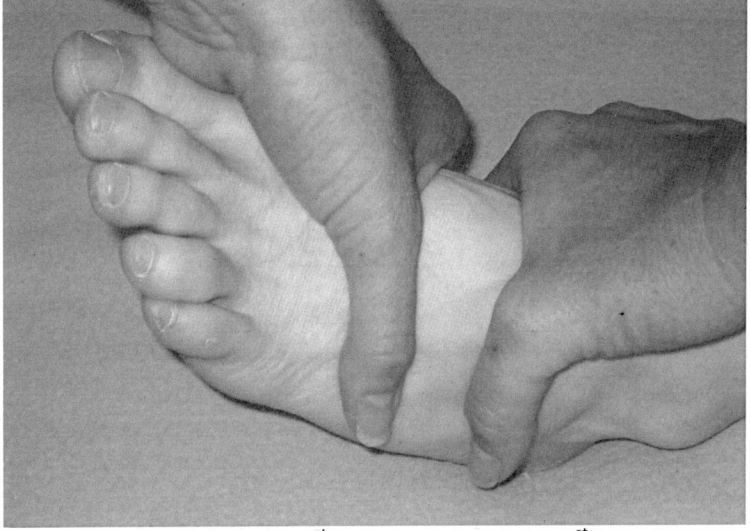

Fig. 9.22   Holding the 1ˢᵗ metatarsal and the 1ˢᵗ cuneiform

Toes

Hold the toes! Place thumb and index (or middle, or fourth) finger on either side (top and sole) of the first phalange of the big toe. Compress and release.

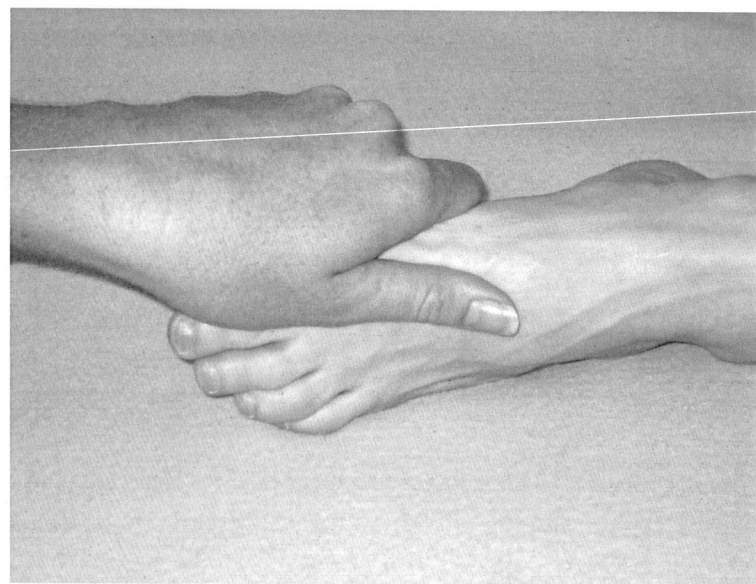

Fig. 9.24

Holding the 1st (the big) toe

Move to the first phalange of the second toe. Compress and release. Repeat across all five toes.

Move to the second phalange of the big toe. Compress and release. Repeat across all toes until all the phalanges have been relaxed.

Note: The toe joints may move very quickly, and the movements, if any, are usually *very* small. I usually only spend a few seconds assessing each toe unless there is something clearly wrong in a toe joint. If there is a problem with a specific toe, then spend extra time and attention on that one spot. In general, the toes will be responsive and will not even require much holding. Hammertoes and other toe contortions are very often caused by tensions a *good distance away* from the toes: the problem may be coming from the cuneiforms or even the ankle joints. Some of the worst hammertoes I've ever seen have been resolved by working on the ankles – not on the toes.

Sometimes hammertoes relax in response to work done on the *center* of the foot: sometimes hammertoes don't relax until the *ankles* relax. I've *never* seen them relax due to working on the toes themselves.

Repeat the above toe sequence with the thumb and finger-of-choice on either side (medial and lateral) of each toe, going over every phalange.

You can go over the foot many times. You can hold the bones in the ankle-to-toes sequential order suggested above or in whatever order you feel like, several times. If some stubbornly held place does release in response to your holding, it is very likely that some

94

other previously stuck joint articulation may now be able to move. The bones are assembled somewhat like those old wooden ball puzzles in which the pieces are so curiously interconnected that you cannot really move any puzzle piece until you figure out which one to move first. Sometimes it may seem as if no bones will move until they are all ready to move. On each pass over the foot, each bone may make scarcely perceptible adjustments even when you are doing nothing but quickly assessing. At some point, all of the bones may have corrected their own position enough so that suddenly they will *all* move smoothly and easily.

On the other hand, while working your way across the foot and ankle, it is very likely that you will come across one or several locations that feature such supreme rigidity that you can safely assume that this area wants something deeper.

This area probably wants the resting-in-one-place-for-a-long-time type of holding: the FSR that we do on injuries from which a person has dissociated.

Finish going over the foot, making your assessments, and then, returning to the place that seemed to want the most work, sit back, get comfortable, and apply the "no motion, no nudging, no intention" type of FSR in the location that needs it. Or, if you prefer, you may stop the assessment process right when you find an "obvious" place that needs holding, and settle in.

Which shall it be? Stop exploring and just hold the place where you detect a stubborn problem, or keep going and come back to it later? You decide. Follow your intuition.

Neither sequence nor timing for "correct" FSR is carved in stone

You truly can approach the sequence and timing of the leg-to-foot FSR in whatever manner seems best to you, according to the silent instructions that you are receiving from your patient's leg.

A frequent remark from practitioners who come to observe members of the PD Team can be paraphrased this way: "I think I'm starting to get it; I've seen five of you doing FSR, and you're all doing exactly the same thing, but you're all doing it so differently! And when I watched one of you in particular working on the same patient that you'd worked on a week earlier, you approached his leg completely differently the second time."

A teaching video: an aside

Although many people have asked for a video or DVD of someone practicing the following technique, it would be pointless: there is nothing to see. A video of me holding someone's ankle to see if there was a subtle responsiveness would just show, to the observer, footage of me sitting motionless, with my hands motionless, on a person's motionless ankle. I might sit there for several minutes or an hour, not doing anything, waiting for the ankle to respond. This would be supremely boring. Again, there would be nothing to see.[1]"

---

[1] One time, years ago, I bowed to popular demand and made a video of myself holding a person's leg, ankle, and foot in various holding positions. I spoke into the microphone very clearly, stating that I was *not* actually doing FSR. FSR is very slow and boring to watch. Instead, I was merely placing my hands on the subject's leg, ankle and foot in order to demonstrate some of the possible holds that a person might want to try. I moved fairly quickly through the various hand poses, stating over and over that I was just demonstrating a sampling of hand positions in order to help people get started who might otherwise be shy about putting their hands on someone's foot; I was not doing FSR. (Continued on next page.)

The next photos are merely for review: they show some basic hand positions for holding the intermediate cuneiform bone – a place where you will probably spend most of your time if you are treating a person with Parkinson's or a person with a mid-foot injury.

Basic foot holding position, with focus on the cuneiform bones: three pictures

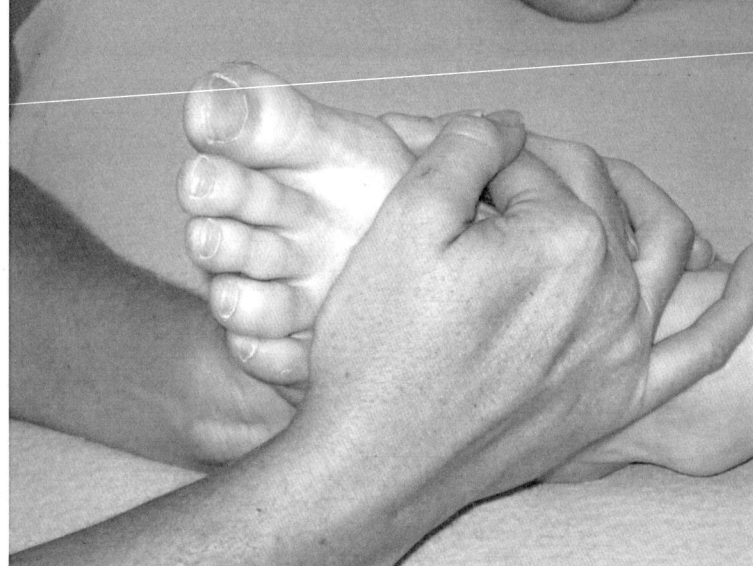

Fig. 9.23

Holding the intermediate cuneiform

(Continued from previous page.) After I released the video, I got many complaints from patients: previous to seeing the video, their therapists, working only from my book, had been going nice and slow, feeling their way along the legs and feet of their patients, spending as much time at each location as was necessary to bring about relaxation. But *after* seeing the video, the therapists had copied the *tempo* of my videoed hand movements. Just as I had quickly moved from one position to another, the therapists were now moving their hands quickly from one spot to another. In other words, the visual cues from the video were too compelling; the spoken instructions on the video were completely ignored.

If I ever release another video, it will be the most boring thing on earth. In it, I shall demonstrate the tempo at which I go when a person's legs do not respond at all: I shall set my hands down in one place and hold them there for a solid minute or two, maybe half an hour. Any nudging or movement on my part would, correctly, be so small as to be invisible.

Then I will go to the next holding position and hold my hands there for half an hour. It will take an hour before the viewer has seen the merest fraction of all the possible ways that a practitioner might want to set his hands down on his patient. It will be so boring, no one will watch more than a few minutes of it before he is saying, "Enough already! Just show me the various hand positions, I understand that I am supposed to go slowly."

But I will not be fooled this time into thinking that this attempt will be different: too many people will *not* understand. Also, every patient is different. Each patient might need to have his foot bones held from a slightly different position and for a different amount of time.

People usually follow visual images more exactly than they follow words. The whole point of FSR is that the practitioner has to learn to follow his hunches and respond to the patient, not to a video. So I suspect that there will not be another foot-hold video in my future.

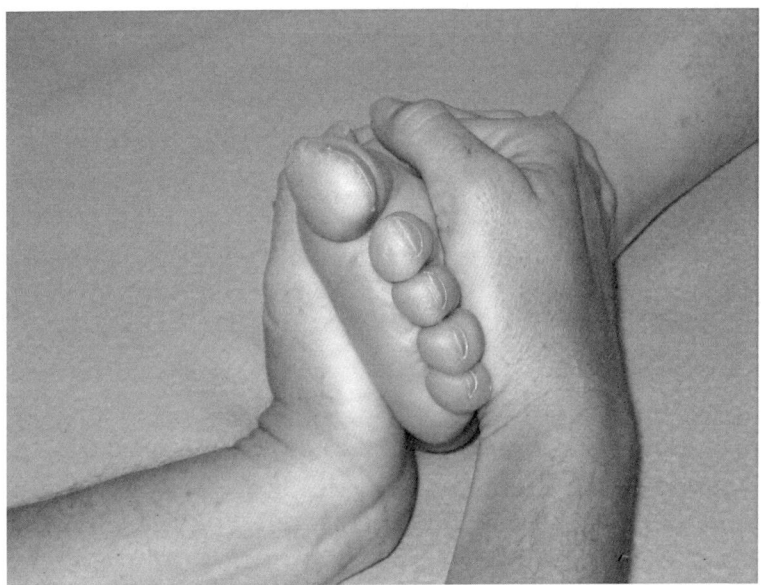

Fig 9. 24

Holding the intermediate cuneiform. The palm of the hand is flush on the sole of the foot, same as the previous photo, but viewed from a different angle.

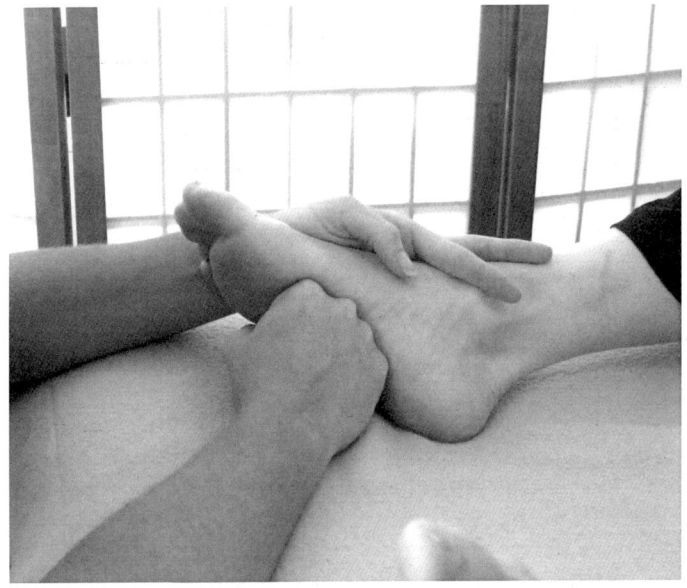

Fig. 9.25

view #3 a variation: the back of the hand flush on the sole of the foot

As you can see, either the palm or the back of the hand can be used. It makes no difference. The important thing is to be able to give a feeling of complete, full support to the bottom and top of the foot.

This chapter has shown many examples of ways that you can hold someone's foot. Please do not think that you must place your hands in any or all or the positions shown above. It is better to just place your hands where they feel like they are supporting whatever area seems to need support, based on that area's inability to relax and be responsive.

Important

Before the publication of this book, a much shorter, five-chapter description of FSR for Parkinson's was available on line. These chapters had no photographs whatsoever – only text descriptions of the basic concepts, short descriptions of some possible hand positions, and a few pen and ink drawings of holding the forearm.

Working from these simple text descriptions, having no photos to "follow," many people with no bodywork experience whatsoever were able to master the FSR enough so that their PD patient recovered. It is simple, supportive holding, such as anyone would intuitively do for any injured person, if they had not learned the cultural restrictions that make us afraid of touching. Holding an injured person is *not* rocket science.

The following was excerpted from an email from someone I've never met. She was working from the photo-less, short-version instructions on doing FSR for Parkinson's. It demonstrates my point:

"Thank you. I am sitting here crying with relief. I don't want to inundate you with emails but I think you may be interested in what happened last night. I have lacked confidence in my ability to hold my husband's foot properly and in the end I just had to trust, although I had not been doing very much. The last two nights I have spent about an hour holding, sometimes falling asleep while I am doing it. Last night I got the usual tingling sensation but stronger and having worked my way down his leg I was holding his foot. (He has been telling me that he had experienced leg twitching after one holding session so I took that as a good sign.)

"Last night when I reached his foot the sensation was very strong. I saw in my mind an ice blue light in his foot and then he literally leaped off the bed as if he had been given an electric shock. He did not wake up.

"I didn't say anything to him because I did not want to influence any response and he told me, unprompted, that he felt looser and more flexible. Then I told him what had happened. His face looked more healthy to me this morning and he adjusted his posture to something so close to normal. The angle of his head and neck was a miracle to see.

"...Thank you... We will continue on our own for now but I don't feel alone or unsupported anymore..."

This person was obviously doing a great job of holding her spouse's foot. She was not working from photographs, or any visual cues. She was not sure of herself. But she just started holding his foot, and his foot came back to life.

So don't follow the photos too closely. They are just suggestions. At some point, within the first session or the second, you should put this book aside and stop thinking about "technique" and just enjoy yourself. The most important thing to remember is support, support, support.

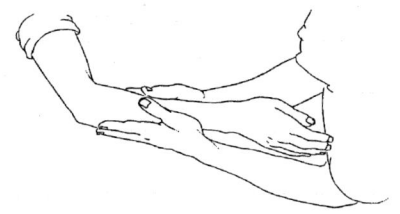

Chapter ten

Testing the feet

Apply some tests! While a foot's ability to move in the directions described below is not a 100% guarantee that blockages are loosening up, it can be a fairly good indication that things are going the right way.

A healthy reflex

The foot has a wonderful reflex that it can do only when all of the bones in the foot are gliding across their articulations freely and easily. The reflex can be triggered with the following stimulation:

The patient should be lying down on a treatment table with straight legs. Place one hand over the patient's foot, with the center of the palm placed on the top, or dorsum of the foot, directly *over* the intermediate cuneiform bone. The rest of the hand can rest on the top of the foot wherever it's comfortable. Then, place your other hand, in a fist position, on the *sole* of the foot, *under* the intermediate cuneiform bone.

Press the hands together slightly and then release. This use of the word "press" refers to an actual, physical compression, one that's visible to the naked eye. The press should be quickly followed by relaxation.

This pressing and relaxing is a *significant* movement, as opposed to the mental, infinitesimally small nudges and pulsing movements that you've used up until now. You are doing this to initiate a reflex muscle movement in the foot.

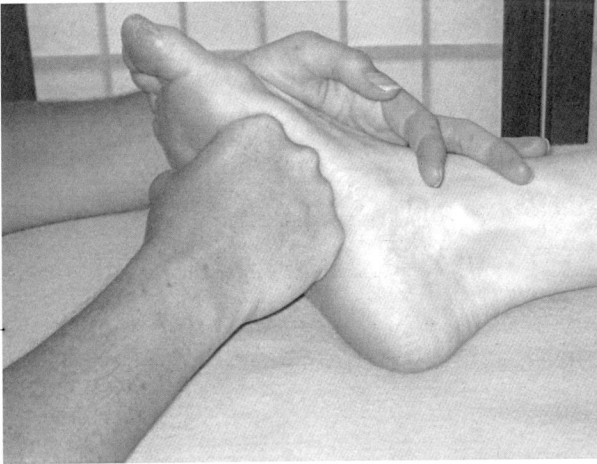

Fig.10.1 Gently punching the foot, looking for a reflexive movement

Your hands should remain on the foot during the subsequent reflexive movement, if any. The foot, if its bones are all in the correct position and unhampered by tensions may, in response to being very gently punched on the sole of the foot, reflexively relax in one of two directions. The two reflexive foot movements are these:

1. The foot may stretch out as if the toes are being pointed like a ballerina. The center line of the top of the foot will straighten out, forming a straight line which is a continuation of the tibial crest. (Fig. 10.2)

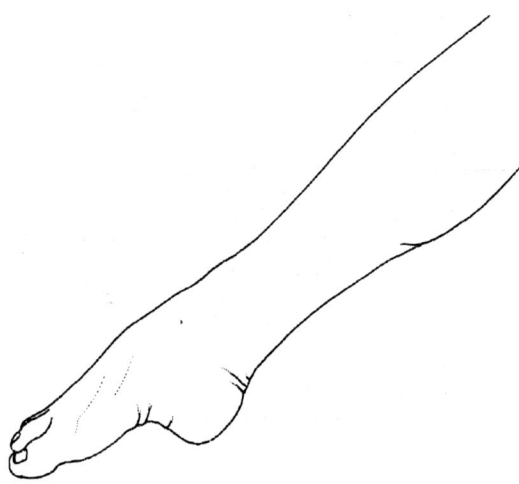

Fig. 10.2   A straight line from leg to toes

A completely relaxed foot, when pushed quickly and gently in the arch area, might easily go into a pointed-toe position. If the ankle is *also* aligned correctly, the ridge of the tibial crest to the center of the foot will form a nice, almost straight line. If there is a problem in the ankle area, the ankle joint may form a concave dip instead of making a nice smooth line.

If a PD patient is doing very well, he will at some point be able to form this pointed toe posture on his own, without needing to be pushed in the arch.

2. The foot may rotate, causing the toes to form a line that is perpendicular to the floor. The big toe will be the toe which is farthest from the surface of the table. The line from the big toe through the little toe forms the perpendicular line. (See Fig. 10.4.)

In the starting position, the right foot is pointing towards the ceiling, and midline of the right foot is more or less in a straight line with the knee. (The right foot appears to be

102

pointing forward more than the left foot. This is because the right foot has been held for a bit, and is more relaxed.) Fig. 10.3.

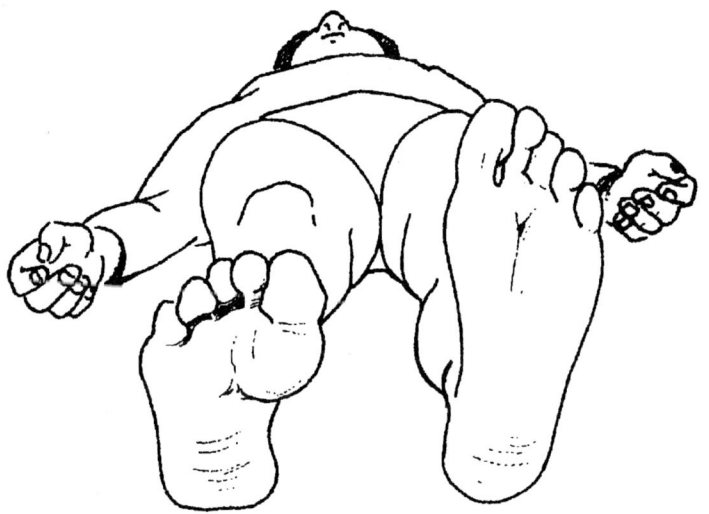

Fig. 10.3

After being bumped gently but firmly in the arch, the right foot may respond, if it is completely relaxed and flexible, by rotating laterally (out to the side). (Fig. 10.4, below.) The knee will *not* have rotated a considerable distance; the rotation will have come from mostly from the relaxed ankle.

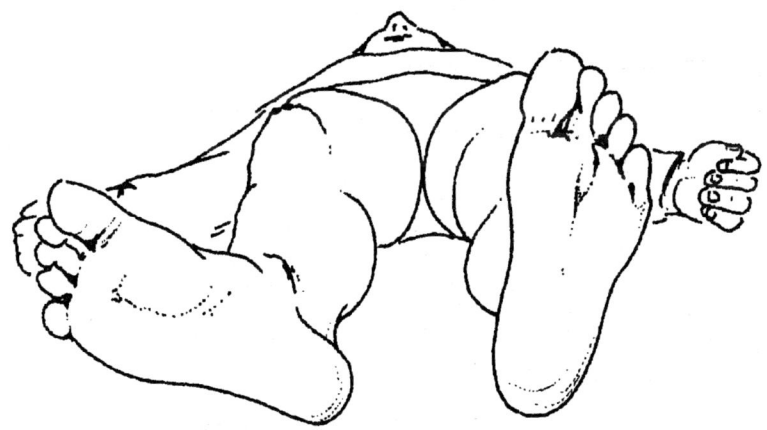

Fig. 10.4 Foot rotation in response to a push on the arch

If the foot articulations are not yet correct, the response to the reflex test may be:
1. The foot will not straighten out (Fig. 10.2), but will remain at more or less of a right angle to the *tibia*.
2. Instead of rotating laterally (Fig. 10.4), a foot that is still injured may reflexively rotate medially, *towards* the arch, as if protecting the arch of the foot instead of exposing it.

Hammer-toes

Also, if displacements or unhealed injuries are present in the ankle and/or foot, the tendons in the foot may pull back on the toes, creating hammer-toes (see Fig.s 10.5 and 10.6).

Hammer-toes are not uncommon in Parkinson's disease. But they are also not uncommon in people who do not – and never will have – PD. Hammer-toes do *not* mean a person is at risk for Parkinson's disease. That having been said, hammer-toes are a sure sign that there is tension or injury somewhere in the foot, ankle, lower leg, knee, or even somewhere upstream from the knee.

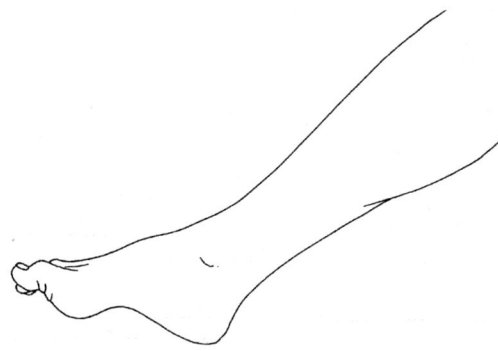

Fig. 10.5
Moderate hammer-toe of the first (big) toe

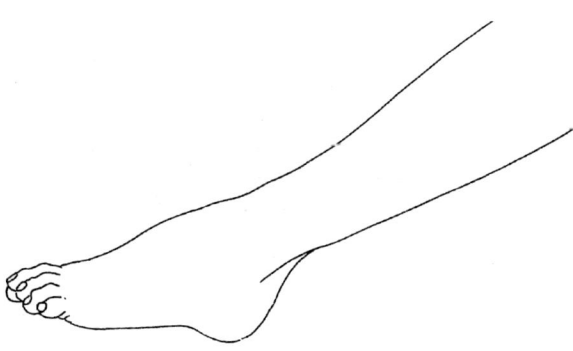

Fig 10.6
Mild hammer-toe of the second toe

If a hammer-toe is present, your work might not be done. The presence of a hammer-toe suggests that the foot is still not fully relaxed. However, patients have recovered from Parkinson's even though their hammer-toes never went away. If his channel Qi has resumed running correctly in his feet, and/or his Parkinson's symptoms are going away, don't worry about the hammer-toe.

I have had PD patients with severe hammer-toes who recovered from Parkinson's even with some residual amount of hammer-toe. Still, some recovered patients worry about their hammer toes. So, I repeat: if your patient has recovered from PD but still has some hammer-toe going on, don't worry about it. Leave it be.

Don't be pushy

Be very careful when you do test the feet to insure that *you are not trying to exert influence over the direction of the foot reflex.*

Do your reflex pulse, and then be a passive observer of which way the foot wants to go. Sometimes it is hard to be impartial; after working for hours on a foot, it is only natural that you will be secretly rooting for the foot to relax straight and long and/or rotate outward. But try not to impose your wishes on that foot. Do a realistic assessment of the reflex. When the foot responds correctly to this test, and the joints all seem to glide smoothly and easily, and there are no areas of the foot that feel somehow less than "correct," you *may* be finished with working on the feet. If so, congratulations.

Flexible feet that still want FSR

But you may not yet be finished working on the feet. The real indication that you are finished is when Qi flows deeply and at full volume through the foot portion of the Stomach channel, and the patient can move his feet normally in all the usual directions, and he can feel his foot moving, and he likes the feeling of moving his foot.

Sometimes, because of residual *emotional* resistance in the injured area, you may not be finished with FSR on the foot in question – even if *you* can move the foot around easily.

Because slow and steady FSR can be an effective way to assist in emotional healing, as well as structural healing, sometimes FSR will still be beneficial even after the foot begins to resume flexibility.

A common question is "How will I know when the foot no longer needs to be held."
Answers: if the person's PD symptoms are gone, you can stop holding.

If *you* can move the patient's foot easily in all the normal directions, but the patient can't move his own feet easily, at will, continue with foot FSR treatments.

If the foot seems healthy and channel Qi flows through the foot but the person still has some areas in his body that are stiff, you might want to start looking for some other unhealed injuries, and apply Yin Tui Na in those areas. (More on this in the next chapter.)

If the foot relaxes sometimes, but tightens up at other times, the patient is dissociating from his heart during those times when the foot it tight. Oppositely, a physiological injury does *not* come and go. Fear and the concomitant heart dissociation *can* come and go – and cause rigidity in the legs and feet when it's present.

If the foot is sometimes relaxed with normal channel Qi flow, and sometimes rigid or having either no channel Qi or backwards flowing channel Qi, it is the patient's thoughts, his dissociation from the heart, and not an injury, that is causing the change ups.

In Chinese medicine, the difference between a problem that comes and goes is differentiated from a problem that is constant, with a fixed location. The former is considered to be a "Qi" problem, or what we might call an energy-*directing* problem. The latter is considered to be a "fixed location, tangible" problem, or, in Chinese, a "Blood Stagnation" problem: a problem that we might call a not-yet-healed physical injury.

If foot rigidity or blockage of energy in the foot comes and goes, the patient must learn to stop dissociating from the heart. The subject of re-associating with the heart is discussed in the book *Recovery From Parkinson's*.

Chapter eleven

Shoulders and hips

Many people with Parkinson's will have unhealed injuries in areas other than just the foot. It is very possible that they have dissociated from these injuries, which is why the injuries have remained unhealed. Sometimes, the patient will volunteer that an area other than the foot also "wants" to be worked on. Usually, you will be looking for other problem areas if the patient has pain or unusual stiffness in that area, or if you have noticed some rigidity in an area that just doesn't feel right.

If the area is in a non-joint area, such as somewhere along the length of the femur (long bone of the upper leg), then choosing the location of the "holding position" for the health practitioner's hands is simple: simply put a hand on either side of the bone near the area that feels rigid and unresponsive, either top and bottom, or side to side, and then sit there, holding it for as long as it takes to get a response. Simple.

However, if the injury seems to be in a *jointed* area such as the hip or the shoulder, there are a number of ways in which the joint might be held. This chapter will offer a few starter suggestions on ways to hold these more complex areas. Of course, once the practitioner is comfortable with working on joints, he will allow his hands to take the lead in deciding where to be placed.

Shoulder

Have the patient lie on his back, if at all possible. Slide one of your hands under his scapula (shoulder blade).

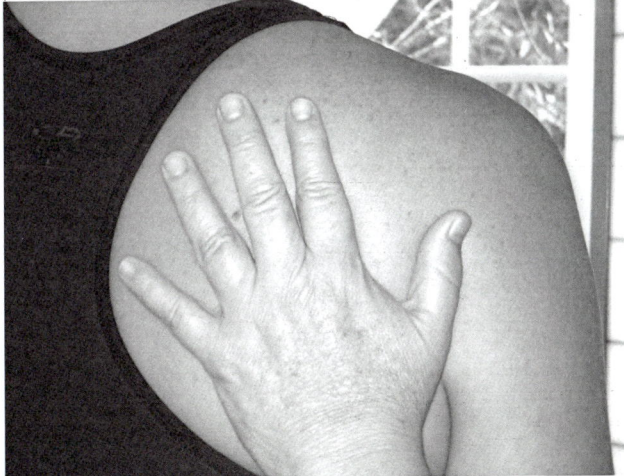

Fig. 11.1 A hand placed on the patient's scapula (shown with patient standing)

Rest your other hand firmly in the depression just below the shoulder edge of the clavicle, on the front side of the body – just above the lung. (Fig. 11.2)

With one hand firmly under the scapula, press down firmly with the clavicle hand and then let up on the pressure. If there is no injury and the joint is relaxable, the scapula will respond to this press by moving medially – towards the spine. If the shoulder area has an injury or is fearful, when you compress the clavicle towards the scapula, the scapula will move laterally – away from the spine – as if trying to rotate around to the front of the body: curling forward as if to protect the injury.

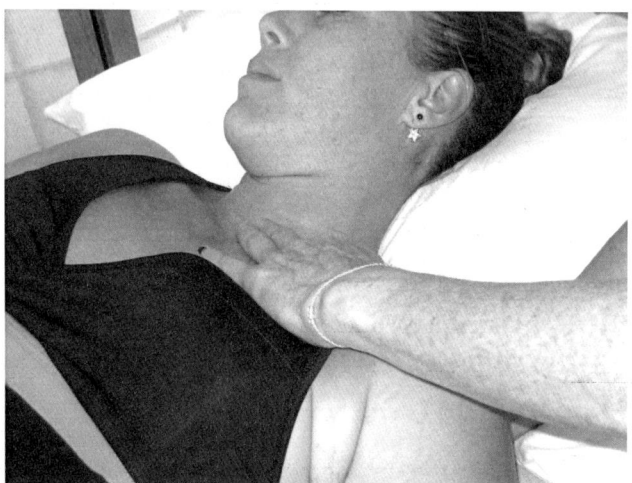

Fig. 11.2 The lower hand on the scapula, upper hand just below the clavicle

If the scapula doesn't move at all, that also suggests a protective, or even dissociated situation in the shoulder and/or overall body.

If the above test, or a visually obvious displacement of anything in the shoulder area, suggests an unhealed injury, consider the following hand positions for your FSR work.

The patient should be lying on his back. Seat yourself facing the patient, at about the level of the patient's shoulder

Place one hand, the hand closest to the person's head, around the "epaulet" area – where the arm inserts into the shoulder socket, and where the lateral end of the clavicle terminates. Get a good, firm grip on this rounded area. (Fig. 11.3)

Place the other hand on the center of the upper-arm bone, the humerus. The best way to position this other hand is to bring it *under* the arm, gripping the side of the humerus that is resting on the table, rather than gripping the humerus from the top (facing the ceiling) side. (Fig. 11.3)

With your hands in these two positions, one cupping the shoulder/top of the arm and the other firmly gripping the humerus, the patient's shoulder joint will feel absolutely supported. Maybe waggle your hands a tiny bit, to show yourself and the patient just how firmly you are supporting the shoulder.

Next, gently nudge, or imagine nudging, the ball at the top of the humerus bone a bit deeper *into* the shoulder socket. Notice if there is a response. Often, the response will seem like the humerus moves away from the socket, in opposition to what you have suggested. So long as any movement response occurs, fine. Go on to the next nudge.

Nudge the humerus as if you are pulling it slightly *out* of the socket. Again, note if a response occurs.

You will now do a series of twelve nudges that will check the responsiveness of all the various muscles and articulations that circle the shoulder. Imagine that a ring around the ball of the humerus is numbered one through twelve, like the face of a clock.

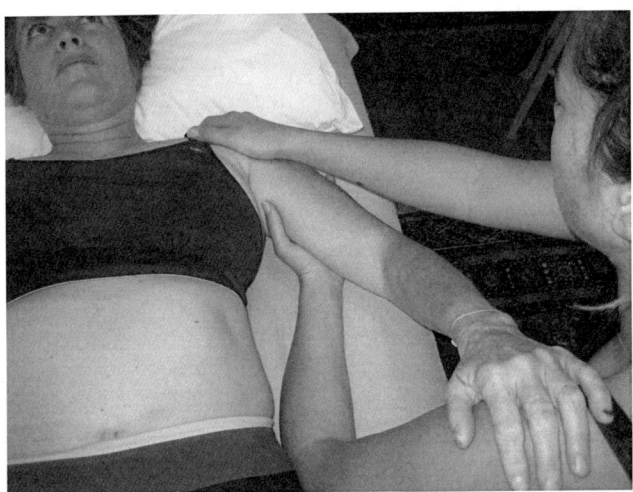

Fig. 11.3   One hand on shoulder, the other holding the humerus.

I usually imagine that the number one is located at the top humerus, just under the acromion (lateral end of the clavicle). The number six is at the bottom of the ball of the humerus, in the armpit. On the right arm, the three is located at the anterior (forward) side of the ball of the humerus, and the nine is located at the posterior (back) side of the ball. On the left arm, the three is posterior and the nine is anterior. This all sounds very fancy but, really, when you sit down and imagine a clock face, it becomes pretty simple and obvious.

The other numbers are placed sequentially around the ball of the humerus, like the numbers on a clock face.

These numbers are mentally superimposed merely to help keep track of the small increments you will nudge in, as you work your way around the shoulder. Once you've mentally got your orienting numbers in place, briefly nudge the humerus upwards, towards the number one and then relax. Notice if there was *any* tiny reaction or movement in the area in response to the nudge.

If so, go on to the number two and give the arm bone a nudge in that direction. If not, do more subtle nudges in the direction of the number one. If, after several nudges, nothing moves, make a mental note to return to this area, and move on to number two, where you repeat the assessment process. And so on, around the "clock."

After making the rounds of the "clock," return to any area that simply refused to respond and settle in for a good long sit, with your hands supporting the shoulder area: one hand cupped over the shoulder and the other hand firmly gripping the humerus. Now and then, as inspired to do so, try again to give a nudge in the direction that was frozen. And now and then, place the hands in the first shoulder testing position, with one hand under the scapula and the other hand in the depression just below the clavicle.

These hand-position suggestions will give you a start at feeling comfortable with "where to put the hands" while working on the shoulder. As you get more familiar with the sensation of working with the shoulder joint, you can feel free to try other holding positions, as well.

And did I mention, you should first try this on a person with healthy shoulders? It is very common to find hang-ups, that is to say, areas that won't budge, on healthy people who have had dislocated shoulder, broken arms, falls from a bicycle, or other arm/shoulder injuries. So do not be discouraged if your practice person turns out to have some areas that don't move. Be pleased! You can go ahead and treat the asymptomatic person, thus preventing a possible painful shoulder situation that might have otherwise crept up in old age.

Hip and leg joint

The hip area is very similar to the shoulder area: the ball of the femur (the femur is the long bone of the upper leg) rotates in the hip socket in very much the same manner that the ball of the humerus rotates in the shoulder socket.

Getting your hands in position to work on the hips

Sit or stand facing the patient, just below the level of the hip. Place one hand under the lateral-distal (lateral means closer to the side, or your might say farther from the spine; distal means closer to the feet, farther from the head) part of the buttock. Elevate the patient's near knee while keeping his near foot flat on the table. Next, using your other arm, bend your shoulder in towards the patient and place your shoulder under the bridge formed by the knee. Bring your hand under the patient's leg and firmly grip the backside or side of the femur.

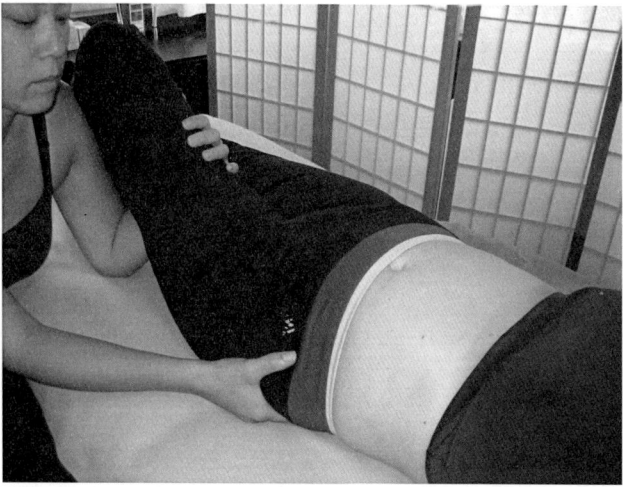

Fig. 11.4   One hand holding the side of the hip, the other holding the leg

I sometimes place the patient's knee up on my shoulder while gripping the leg firmly. This extra support for the patient's leg creates an even stronger illusion that the patient's body is being "fully supported" even though I am only using a very small area of my own body to "control" a fairly large area on the patient.

Now, holding all this area firmly, begin by nudging or imagining nudging the ball of the hip farther into the hip socket.

Next, nudge the ball out from the socket.

Then, just as explained with the ball of the shoulder, imagine a clock face, numbered one through twelve, around the hip joint. I usually put the one at the top (towards the person's head) of the socket, and the six down at the bottom (towards the feet) of the socket. I put three at the back of the socket, and nine at the front, and fill in the rest of the "clock face" accordingly.

Notice if there are any areas that do not respond, and give them extra time, or go back to them later, after you've assessed the whole hip area.

Hips and sacrum

For the novice, getting a good, supportive grip on the back part of the hip joints, the sacro-iliac joint, can be a bit tricky. Where do you even begin? Happily, there are several techniques for getting the hip joint firmly in control of your hands.

The best requires that you be standing up, facing the patient, with the patient lying on his back.

You will start by working on the hip that is farther from you, rather than the closer hip.

Reaching for the patient's farther leg, bring the patient's farther knee up while keeping the patient's farther foot flat on the table. And ask the patient to keep it there while you get your hands in place.

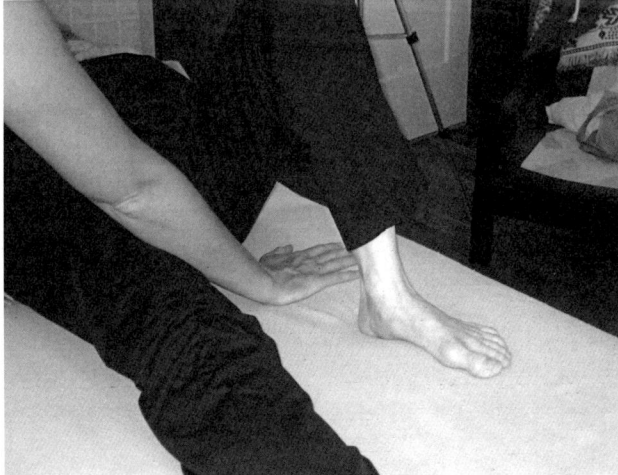

Fig. 11.5 **Place your hand under the "bridge" formed by the patient's farther knee**

Put your arm – the arm closer to the patient's feet, not the arm closer to the patient's head - under the "bridge" formed by the patient's elevated knee. Place your hand, palm down, on the table on the far side of the bridge.

Place your other arm on the "ASIS" (anterior superior iliac spine): the bit of the hip bone that protrudes out the front in very slender people. Get a firm grip on the ASIS, or maybe reaching around the side of the ASIS, so that you can lift the hip on this side slightly off the table. Gently raise the far hip a mere inch or so off the table

Tell the patient to be limp in the hips – don't try to "help" the practitioner by lifting the hip to high in the air. (If the patient is very large, you may need to ask for his help, but remind him to relax after he's put the hip back down.)

While the hip is raised, slide the other hand, the one that is palm down on the table, under the center of patient's far hip – still palm down, on the table.

Once your hand is centered under the patient's buttock, rotate the "palm down" hand so that your hand is "standing" up: the little-finger side is resting on the table, and the thumb-side is raised up, supporting the patient's hip. This hand position will raise the hip a bit farther in the air. Keep rotating this hand quickly and smoothly until it is palm up, and then let the "upper hand" release its lifting hold on the ASIS.

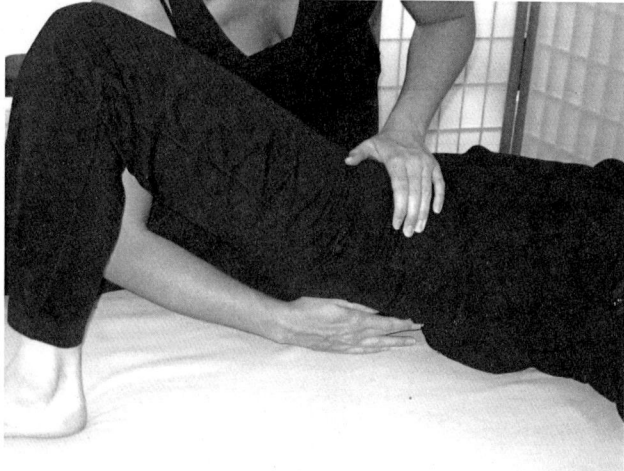

Fig. 11.6 Rotate your hand until it is palm up.

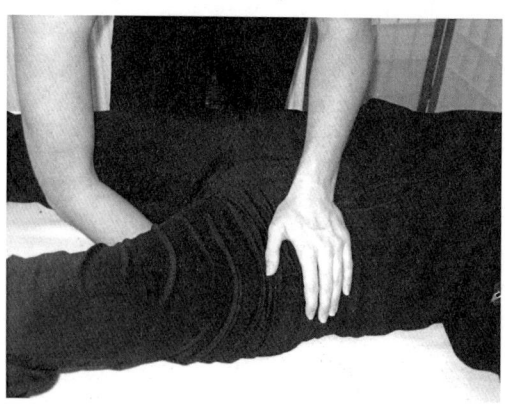

As the patient's hip drops back down to the table, it will automatically settle down in such a way as to minimize the lumpiness of your lower hand. To do this, the patient's body will automatically center itself over your hand, so that you find yourself with your hand directly under the patient's sacrum – the triangular bone at the base of the spine that joins the two hip bones.

Fig. 11.7 Hand under the sacrum

You must practice this move *several* times for it to become smooth and effortless. But once you have mastered it, it is an elegant, quick, and smooth way to position one hand under the sacrum, with no disquieting fumbling in the vicinity of the genitals.

With one hand under the sacrum, you can now place the other hand on the ASIS, which gives you a good starting place to supportively hold while checking on the reflexive movement in the sacro-iliac joint.

Take a moment to imagine the diagonal line of the joint where the far-side of the sacrum meets the far ilium (ilium is singular, ilia is plural. Ili*ac* is the adjective form). I say "far side" because this hand positioning requires that you hold the far hip, rather than the near hip.

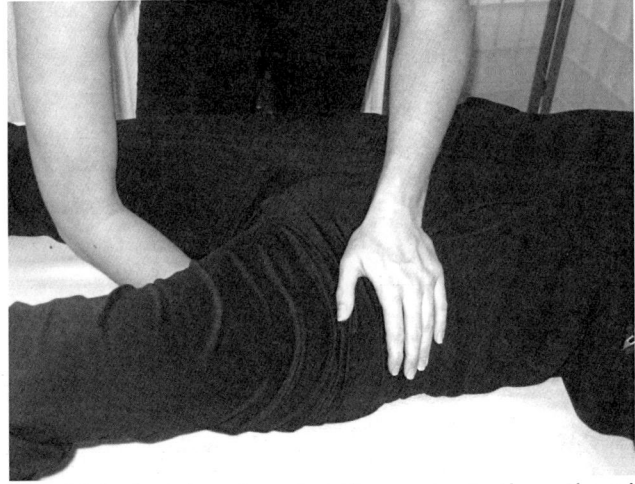

Fig. 11.8 One hand under the sacrum, the other hand on the ASIS, feeling for responsive movement in the sacro-iliac joint

Now you're in position to start nudging, or imagine nudging, that joint.

First, nudge or imagine nudging the joint as if you are compressing the bones more closely together. Remember, these bones meet on a diagonal line. See if there is any response.

Imagine you are moving the bones farther apart.

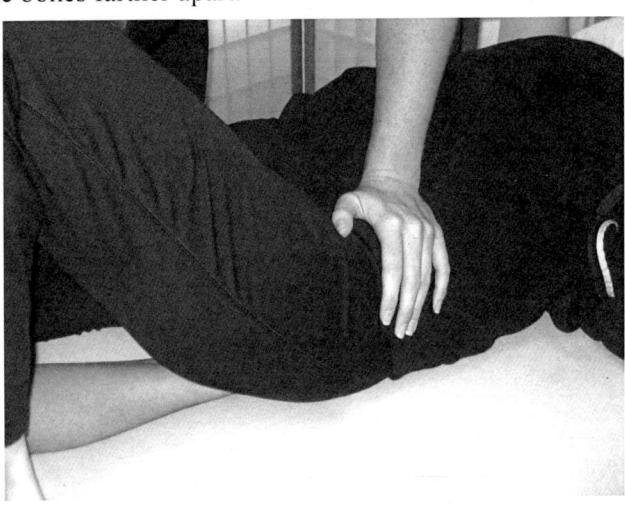

Fig. 11.9 Another view of one hand under the sacrum, the other holding the ASIS

Next, see if the hip bone can move towards the head, relative to the sacrum, which moves towards the feet. Remember, this movement will not be a line that runs parallel to the spine. It is an angled line, so when I say "towards the head" I actually mean "upward, towards the far shoulder." See if there is any response.

Then try moving the ilium in the opposite direction, towards the feet, while the *sacrum* moves towards the head. Again, it is an angled move, not a move that runs parallel to the spine.

Finally, nudge or imagine a nudge that pushes the sacrum ever so slightly forward, towards the front of the body, while nudging the ilium towards the back of the body.

And then the reverse: ilium towards the front, sacrum towards the back.

Remember: all of these moves are extremely subtle. You are not actually moving these bones around. You are merely introducing the slightest of nudges, or even the thought of a movement.

Then, examine/treat the hip on the opposite side of the body: stand on the opposite side of the table and repeat all the above.

This gentle series of moves can sometimes bring about significant relaxation in the hip joints. If some area does not respond to the gentle suggestions, try making the nudge more gentle, or merely imagining it, or try giving the nudge a tiny *bit* more power – but never enough that the patient can tell what you are doing. If the specific nudge still doesn't garner a response, settle in comfortably for a while and just hold the area, keeping firm pressure from your hands as if they are holding the SI joint snugly compressed.

Chapter twelve

The head and spine

The many aspects of head- and spine-holding are worthy of an entire book. In fact, such books have already been written.

If you are going to work on a person's head and spine because you suspect rigidity in those areas or the presence of an unhealed injury, you might do well to buy any of the excellent books already available on the subject of craniosacral therapy.

These books will explain the correct articulations of the skull and spine bones, and suggest the most advantageous placement for the hands.

Of course, these books are just a starting point. Once you get comfortable with your hands on the cranial and spinal bones, you will find that you can branch out on your own, and hold the patient in the places to which your hands are drawn.

You might be able to find a trained craniosacral therapist in your area. But a word of warning: most craniosacral protocols use more force than most Parkinson's patients feel good with. The books on the subject usually suggest using a very low level of force to pull or push the various cranial and spinal bones, in order to encourage them to relax and drift into the most ideal anatomical positions. While many people truly enjoy this gentle pressure, we have found that many, if not most, of our Parkinson's patients find this "low level pressure" to be far too intrusive.

Therapists trained in this modality have been told that the amount of force they need to use is "minimal" or even "imperceptible." But people with Parkinson's will be able to feel these forces and steel themselves against the intrusion. If your local craniosacral therapist can't use an FSR level of patience and non-directed force, you might be better off just doing this work by yourself.

If you are working from a craniosacral instruction book that instructs you to use light force to push or hold in a given direction, don't. Instead, simply place your hands firmly and supportively in the hand positions recommended in the book, and just sit there. Sometimes a very slight directional pressure *might* be appropriate, but generally, for people with Parkinson's disease, the "gentle" forces suggested in the books are too much.

Possibly the best book on the subject is John Upledger's *Craniosacral Therapy*. But be warned, this is a very detailed book, fairly expensive book, and oriented towards health professionals. You don't really need all the theory that he uses to validate his ideas about light touch therapy. All you really need to learn is where to place your hands to best support. So if you don't want to get into a professional level of craniosacral treatment, I've included the following very quick course in hand positions for craniosacral work.

A very quick course in hand positions for craniosacral work.

The following hand positions are usually the most important ones. Of course, once you get familiar with holding the various parts of someone's head or spine, you will be able to branch out on your own. You will let your hands be your guides as to where to hold and support any places on the head or spine that aren't described below. Well-trained craniosacral therapists work in the same way: they learn the basic holding positions, but as they come to get more comfortable working with cranial bones, they branch out on their own and "do what the patient's body tells them to do."

If you are not familiar with the names of the cranial bones, please research the cranial anatomy by going online for more and better pictures than I could hope to include in this book.

I am including photos of the hand positions that can be helpful for holding these areas. Still, for an in-depth understanding of what might move, to where, and why, you might want to read something from the literature that has sprung up around this subject.

Places to hold
1) the occiput
2) the frontal bone
3) the parietal bones
4) the sphenoid bone
5) the sacrum
6) the temporal bones
7) release of diaphragms
8) cervical vertebrae
9) spinal traction

Note: all holding positions assume that the patient is lying down on his back, facing the ceiling.

1. Occiput

Place your cupped hands under the somewhat spherical "ball" of the occiput. You'll notice that, if you sit very still, you might feel the occiput rocking towards you and away from you, as it rocks on the top vertebrae in response to the pumping of the sacrum's

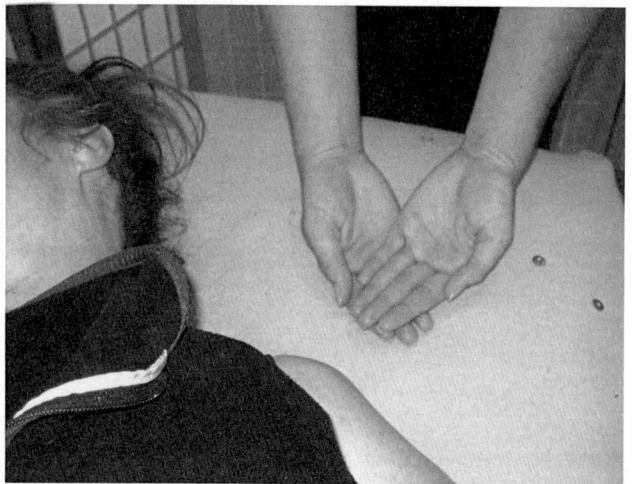

pumping action. This pumping action moves cerebrospinal fluid. Please practice this on a healthy person. People with Parkinson's very often have inhibited flow of cerebrospinal fluid plus rigidity in the neck that can inhibit the pumping motion of the occiput.

Fig. 12.1 Showing how the hands will be positioned when they

are under the head

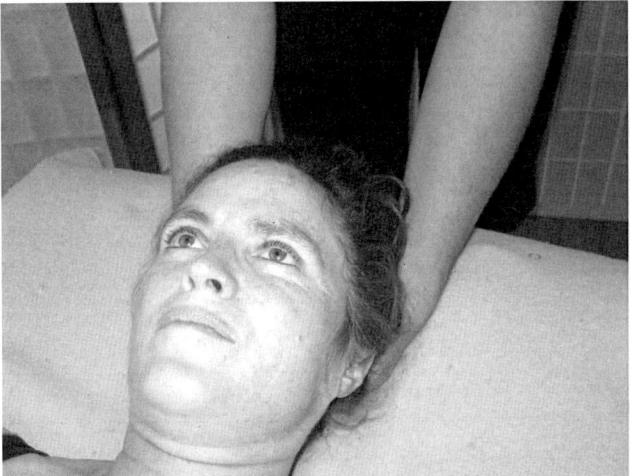

Fig. 12.2 The "cupped" hands seen the in previous photo have been placed under the head, and simply cradle the head. Although this photo shows the therapist standing up, one usually sits while doing this, as you might sit for a long time before the occiput relaxes and begins gently rocking back and forth.

2. Frontal bone

Place your fourth finger, the "ring" finger, on either side of the frontal bone, in the convenient indentation just proximal to the lateral side of the eyebrows. This bone, if relaxed, might be able to move ever so slightly towards the ceiling. If this bone has sustained an injury, it may have become slightly compacted inwards. A movement towards the ceiling will help restore this bone to its correct position. Don't move the bone around. Hold it. Support it. If it *wants* to move, stay with it.

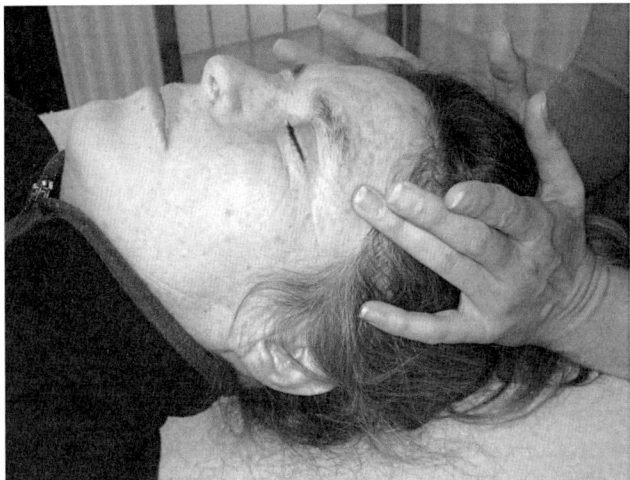

Fig. 12.3 Side view of holding the frontal bone with the 4th finger

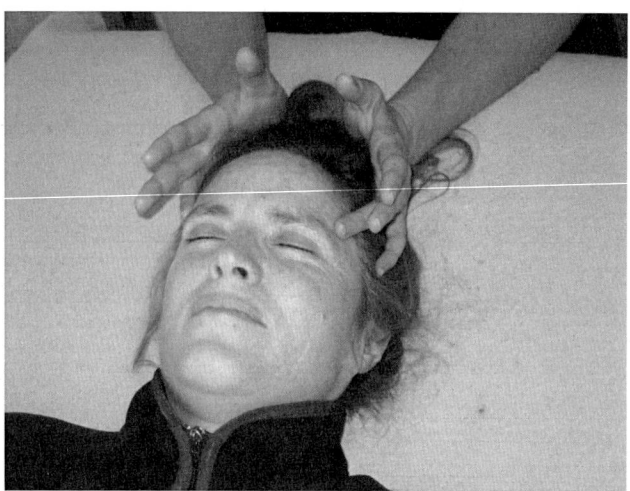

Fig. 12.4 Frontal view of holding the frontal bone with the 4th finger

3. Parietal bones

Place your fingertips where the parietal bones articulate with the temporal bones. These bones articulate with the temporal bones by sliding under the beveled edge of the temporal bones. A blow to these bones can jam them too far down under the edge of the temporal bones. If this happens, the "too tight" parietal-temporal bone articulations can prevent the temporal bones from rotating freely. You may wish to gently *imagine* the parietal bones gently moving towards your own chest as you sit behind the patient's head. This movement will bring the parietals out from under the temporal bones, just a little bit, thus freeing up the temporal bone movements.

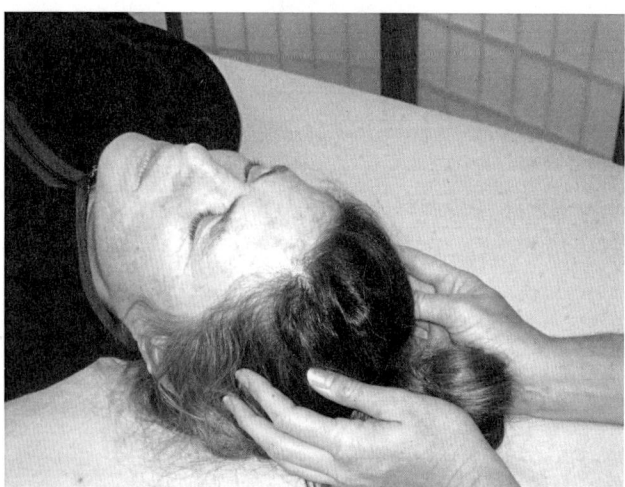

Fig. 12. 5. Holding the parietal bone near the suture (joint) with the temporal bone

118

4. Sphenoid

Rest your thumbs on the sides of the face, just posterior to the eyes, in the small indentation in the skull.

DO NOT nudge these bones in any direction. If you displace the sphenoid bone in the slightest, the person may get a headache, poor visual focus, and other problems. So just rest your thumbs in this spot, making sure you are pushing the sphenoid bone posteriorly, towards the ears.

If the sphenoid bone wants to move of its own accord, allow it to do so. In most cases of sphenoid displacement, the bone has moved too far posteriorly, and will want to move anteriorly, towards the front of the face. But sometimes it needs to move side to side, or one side up and the other side down, or posteriorly.

When I teach craniosacral protocol, the incorrect manipulation of the sphenoid is the one most likely to lead to head problems and complaints from students who've been worked on with too much force, the following day. Be careful with this one.

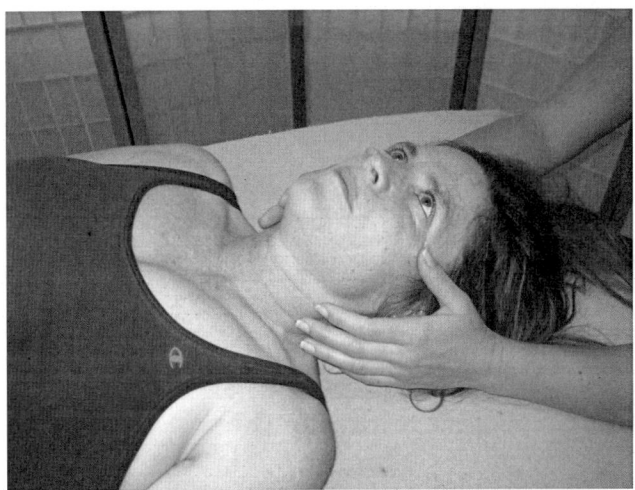

Fig. 12.5 Thumbs resting on the sphenoid bone. In this photo, it almost appears as if the thumbs are pushing towards the jaw – they are not. The thumbs are just sitting, not pushing in any direction.

5. Sacrum

To hold the sacrum, use the same technique described in the previous chapter for getting your hands in the right position to work on the sacroiliac joint. Once you have got your "under" hand positioned nicely under the patient's sacrum, place your upper hand on the patient's abdomen, as close to the pubic bone as you and the patient feel comfortable with. Rest a bit with your hands in this position, and maybe nudge your hands closer together a few times. Support in this position can sometimes allow muscles in the pelvic floor to relax, which then allows the sacrum to position itself more correctly.

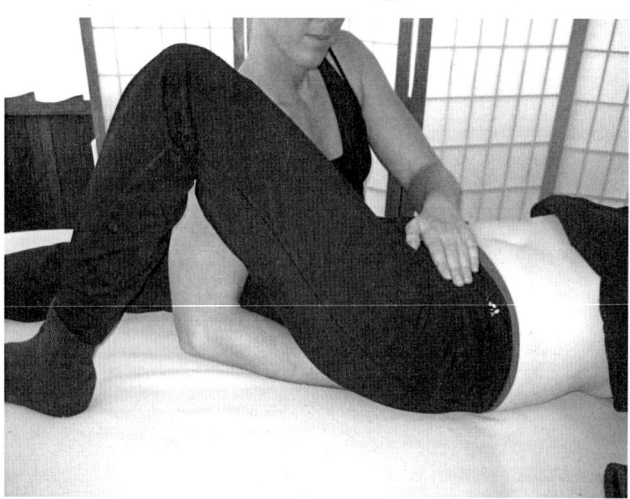

Fig. 12.6 One hand under the sacrum, the upper hand on the abdomen, approaching the pubic bone

6. Temporal bones

Place your fingers in a "circle" around the ear bone – not on the ear itself. Your fingers will need to be "under" the ear, or you might say, resting on the skin of the skull, so that you can get your fingers as close to the center of the temporal bone as possible.

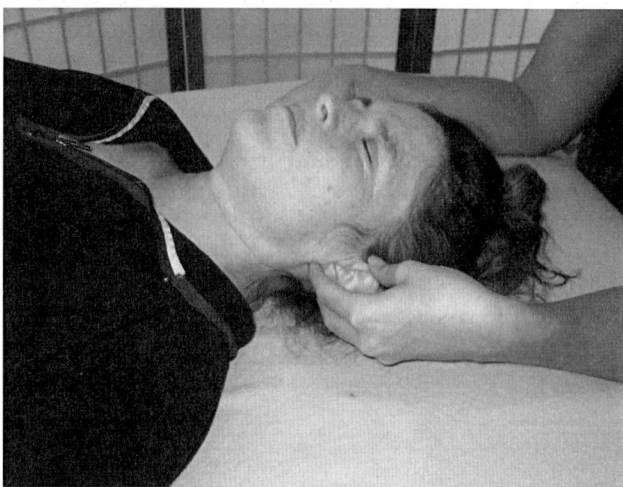

Fig. 12.7 Fingers on the temporal bone: the skin under the ear

With your hands in this position, you might be able to every so slightly rotate the skin over the temporal bones around the axis of the ear hole. If you imagine the somewhat round temporal bone as being the face of the clock, you should be able to move the skin over the temporal bones ever-so-slightly clockwise and counterclockwise. Never use force – if the skin over the ears doesn't want to rotate, then just imagine a rotation.

The temporal bones evolved from our gills. Like gills, they move in a pumping motion, with every breath.

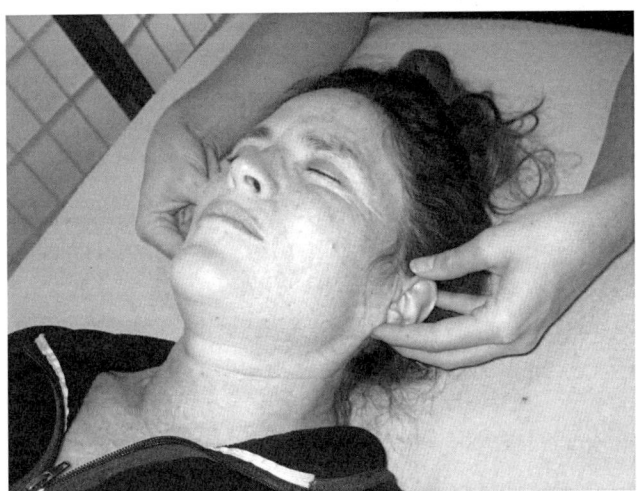

Fig. 12.8 Another view of holding the temporals

In a healthy person with no muscle spasms in the head or spine, the temporal bones rotate slightly backwards with every exhalation, and forward with every inhalation. In this case, "backwards" means "the right ear moves counter-clockwise if you are standing on the patient's right side, looking at the right ear, and the left ear moves clockwise." Another way of thinking of it is that top (proximal, closer to the top of the head) part of the temporal bones moves towards the back of the head with each inhalation, and the bottom of the temporal bone moves towards the chin.

This bone often gets stuck via muscle spasm if a person has a spasm in the psoas muscle, in the back. Even a slight psoas muscle spasm will pull the spine to the side. In order to keep one's eyes level with the ground, a deep, subconscious instinct, a person with spasm in the psoas muscle will usually, without realizing it, choose to use a spasm of the opposite-side temporal bone muscles to make the eyes stay level. This can cause mild headache and is also the number one cause of ear ringing.[1]

7. Diaphragms

Two muscular "diaphragms" might be holding tension: one is under the lungs, the other is the group of muscles at the top of the lungs, bottom of the throat.

---

[1] If you have a patient with recent-onset ear-ringing, you can usually get rid of it in one or two sessions by first getting rid of the psoas muscle spasm, and then teaching the patient how to manually rotate his temporal bones in tune with inhalation. Have the patient place his hands on his own temporal bones and gently rotate them backwards while exhaling. He should do this three times in a row, several times a day. If the ear ringing has been going on for weeks, months, or years, it may take several weeks or months for the patient's body to completely unlearn the habit of spasm in the temporal bone. Also, the patient's psoas spasm must be released. The psoas-spasm release technique is discussed in the next chapter.

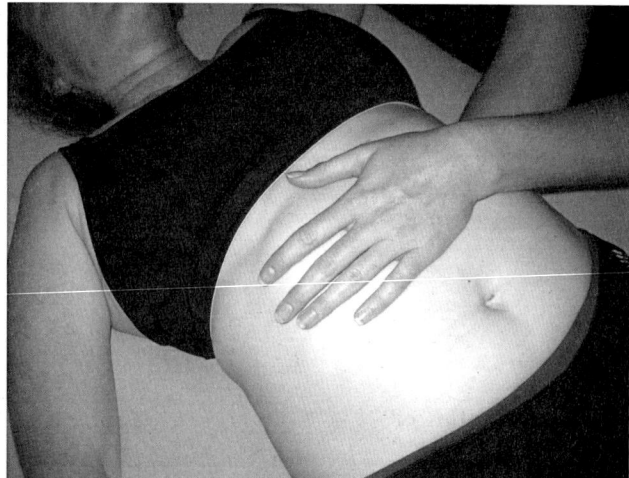
Fig. 12.9 Holding the diaphragm that works the lungs

To release tension in the diaphragm below the lungs, place one hand below the sternum and the other hand under the spine, just below the upper hand. Hold for a bit, and maybe nudge the hands together for a split second, to see if the muscles between your hands can relax. As always, if there is movement, keep your hands in good contact and follow the movement with your hands, maintaining the support.

The next "diaphragm," or collection of muscles that makes a circle, is around the top of the rib cage: the thoracic inlet. Place one hand on the top of the sternum and the other hand underneath the first hand.

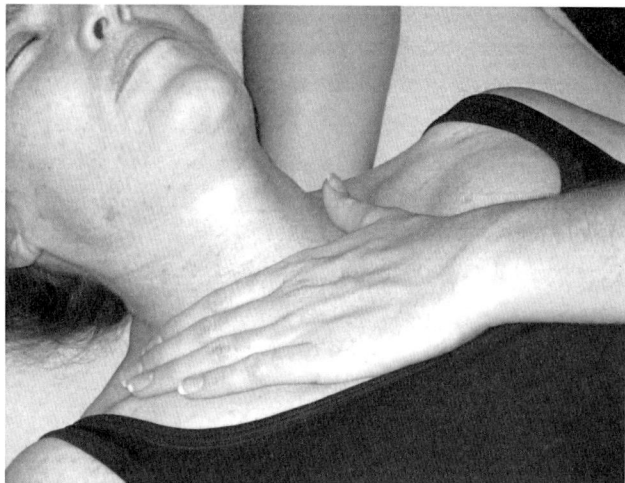
12.10 Holding the thoracic inlet

8. Cervical vertebrae
Place your hands gently on either side of the patient's neck, and just hold. Do not try to move or "adjust" anything! The articulations of these bones are very delicate, and you can

do real and lasting harm by trying to interfere with these bones. This is a book for do-it-yourselfers, as well as medical students. Unless you are medically licensed to move these bones, do not do so. However, just placing your hands on either side of the neck can very often give enough support so that the neck bones, if slightly out of place or the muscles, if slightly in spasm, will move and relax back into their correct places.

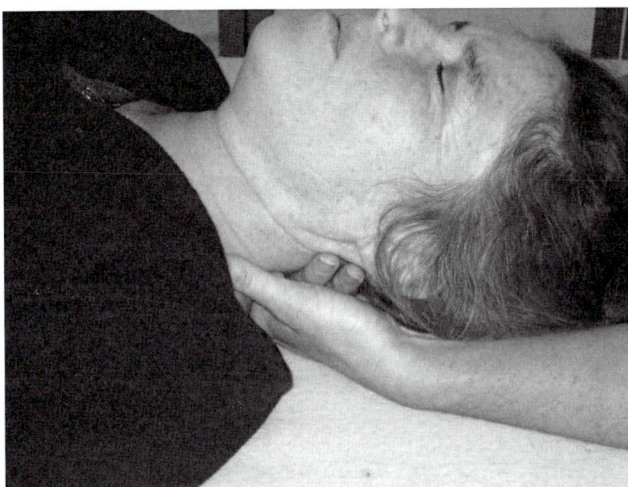

Fig. 12.11 Holding the neck (cervical vertebrae)

9. Spinal traction

Placing one hand under the patient's sacrum, as shown earlier, very, very, very gently *imagine* that you are pulling the sacrum towards the feet. You can imagine that the spine is loosening at each vertebra. You can even count the five lumbar, twelve thoracic, and seven neck vertebrae as you imagine that each one, in turn, is gently moving towards the feet, creating a tiny distance between each vertebrae, one at a time. Even if you only *imagine* that you are pulling the sacrum towards the feet, the patient may feel a genuine lengthening of the spine, and may feel much taller after this treatment.

Oppositely, if you actually pull hard on the patient's spine, he may well tighten up in his spine, to resist you.

Next, while sitting at the head of the table on which the patient is lying, so that you are behind the patient's head, with the top of the patient's head facing you, place your hands on either side of the patient's head, and *imagine* that you are pulling the head oh-so-slighly off of the topmost vertebra by pulling the patient's head towards your chest. Then, continue to imagine the stretch continuing down the patient's spine, going past the seven cervicals, the twelve thoracics, and the five lumbar vertebrae, until your reach the sacrum.

At this point, if your focus has migrated, with your imagination, all the way down to the sacrum, you might be even able to feel the gentle back and forth movement in the sacrum, as it pumps the cerebrospinal fluid.

In all of the above holding positions, place your hands on the patient gently, and remove your hands gently. If the patient's body seems to be magnetically pulling on your hands, then sit with your hands in that position until the patient "lets go" of you, and then gently, respectfully, remove your hands.

It's OK to go to a professional

The above information is not meant to imply that anyone can and should feel comfortable performing craniosacral therapy on friends and loved ones. The above information has been provided because some Parkinson's patients have head, spine, and neck injuries from which they have dissociated *and* they do not live anywhere near a professional craniosacral therapist. For these people, the above, introductory, modified craniosacral therapy holding positions have been provided.

If you live in an area where craniosacral therapists are easy to find (look on the internet, or in your Yellow Pages under massage therapist, acupuncturist, or chiropractor), I highly recommend you use their services.

However, you must let them know right from the beginning that your PD patient finds the "extremely light pressure" that is standard to be too intrusive. Ask the practitioner to just place his hands in the usual positions for the standard protocol and keep them there for a while, in each of the positions, holding firmly, and noticing if the bones spontaneously do any moving on their own.

If the bones do move, great. But if there are areas that, to the experienced hands of the craniosacral therapist, feel "stuck," ask him to either just sit there at those positions, not moving, or else show you which hand positions elicited no response, or a "stuck" response.

Then, you can go home and practice holding these particular areas for an hour at a stretch, which may be what your patient actually needs in order to release in these areas.

If your craniosacral therapist responds to your request by saying, "I don't need to modify my technique: I only use a little pressure to help things move around. It won't be a problem." then ask for a referral to a different craniosacral therapist. Or let the cransiosacral therapist do a few sessions on the patient while you take notes regarding the hand positions – and then go home and practice those hand positions with *no* overt moving of the craniosacral bones – and see which form of treatment your patient prefers.

I've had PD patients who have seen craniosacral therapists who used "minimal pressure or "only five grams of pressure." Some of these patients have felt threatened enough by that "little bit of pressure" that they could feel themselves locking down *more* rigidly or defensively than normal in order to deal with the impositions of the craniosacral therapist. The PDers who feel this way just can't help it: their strong desire to not be "messed with" is stronger than their desire to relax.

If the craniosacral therapist cannot understand this, then find someone else.

As an aside, I very strongly recommend that all my Yin Tui Na students take a professional craniosacral class. After taking a weekend craniosacral class, my Yin Tui Na students who've already spent a few months working on a few PD patients invariably report back to me saying things like, "The other students in the craniosacral class ("other students" referring to those who'd never learned FSR or worked on a person with Parkinson's) were really having a hard time feeling the subtle rhythms and cerebrospinal fluid movements, they kept asking what it was they were looking for. They were having a really hard time feeling *anything*. But it was so *easy* for all of us who've had the Yin Tui Na class. Heck, those cerebrospinal movements were overt, *glaring*, compared to the tiny movements, or the utter non-responsiveness, of our Parkinson's patients!"

In other words, by working with PD patients via sitting for an hour at a time feeling next-to-nothing, by patiently supporting these patients with practically rigid bodies, my students had become so much more "tuned in" to subtle changes and rhythms that the so-called "subtle" and "barely discernable" movements of basic craniosacral therapy were, to them, obvious. And the amounts of pressure that they were instructed to use, in these classes, seemed to my students to be almost offensive. They felt that the supportive, un-intrusive holding that they had been learning in Yin Tui Na class was far more appropriate than the "gentle" amounts of pressure advocated by their craniosacral teachers.

Since I took my first craniosacral class back in the early 1990s, gentler forms of craniosacral therapy have been "invented." There are now several schools of craniosacral therapy that teach the extremely non-invasive, nothin' but holding methods that we use in treating the foot injuries of people with Parkinson's. Still, it seems that the majority of craniosacral therapists study the "gentle pressure" methods – which is far too much intrusion for many people with Parkinson's.

Most practitioners of manual therapy, looking over the extensive scale of body work, ranging from vigorous and manipulative all the way to subtle and gentle, consider craniosacral work to be at the extreme far end of gentle.

But FSR, which very often ends up consisting of holding, doing "nothing at all," is even more gentle. And sometimes, "doing nothing at all" is the only way to unlock the fear and dissociation that has kept an area shut down for decades.

Massage therapists

On paper, FSR sounds easy: hold firmly and don't do anything, and don't impose your thoughts on the patient. But it can be very, very difficult to do this.

Curiously, in my experience, the people who've had the hardest time mastering Yin Tui Na have been the professional massage therapists. Within a few minutes of supportively holding, they want to get busy "doing something."

Several of them have complained to me with something along the lines of, "How can I justify getting payment for not *doing* anything?"

No matter how many times I point out to them that, by firmly holding and remaining motionless for long periods of time, they are providing a very rare and skilled service, one that many people with unhealed injury desperately need, they are still unsatisfied.

They have been trained to push and shove. And unless they are allowed to push and shove, some massage therapists, though not all, feel that they aren't doing anything worthwhile.

So if you are planning to look for a health professional to learn FSR or other forms of Yin Tui Na on your behalf, do not *assume* that just any massage therapist will be your best bet.

On the other hand, some excellent Yin Tui Na therapists have come from the ranks of massage therapists who *do* understand the power of supportive, non-invasive contact.

And then again, ultimately, supportive holding of an injured person is one of the most basic of human instincts. Almost all of us know to hold an injured or frightened infant or young child closely, in a snug embrace. And most of us know how to tell when the infant or child no longer needs to be held.

You do *not* need to be a health professional to learn these techniques and quickly master them. You just need to be willing to go slowly and patiently, without getting emotionally involved in "how fast" the patient is going to heal, or whether or not you are "doing it" correctly. After all, if you are "doing" anything, you are doing too much. Hold the patient firmly, and let him come, in his own time, to his own conclusions about whether or not he feels safe enough to start paying attention to, and *feeling*, his injury, pain, and fear.

Chapter thirteen

Psoas muscle release

A spasm in the psoas muscle is a very, very common occurrence. The majority of back pain problems and sacroiliac problems have their origin in psoas muscle spasm.

The psoas is one of the largest muscles in the body. It attaches to the spine up by the lung's diaphragm, and connects, at the other end, at the top of the femur, the large bone of the upper leg.

The ideal use of this muscle is raising the thigh. Tightening this muscle is said to "decrease the angle of the upper leg and torso."

For example, if you are standing up straight, the "angle" of the torso junction with the thigh is 180°. When your thigh is raised, such as when you are sitting, the angle is decreased to approximately 90°.

Hurting your back

The problem in humans is that they tend to use the psoas muscle to bend forward. This motion also decreases the angle between the torso and thigh: the job of the psoas muscle. However, this muscle was never designed to lever the whole mass of the torso and head. In quadrupeds, this muscle is designed to lift the leg: in a quadruped, the leg is a small percentage of the overall body.

In humans, we might bend forward by tightening the psoas, but the torso and head is a *large* percentage of the overall body in a human. The psoas muscle can over-react to the job, tightening up too much, and going into spasm – from which it doesn't automatically release. If we are leaning even a bit to one side or the other, one side's psoas muscle will tighten more than the other side – and go into spasm, pulling the back violently to one side. When it does this, the nerves that emerge from between the vertebrae can get painfully squeezed: "back pain."

Sometimes, the sacrum even gets pulled to one side by the power of the psoas muscle. In these cases, the nerves in the sacrum can get squeezed (overstimulated), causing a pain sensation that might seem to originate anywhere from the hip to the toe. But even if the pain sensation seems to be coming from the hip or the toe, the actual location of the problem is usually in the psoas muscle. If the psoas muscle can be made to relax, the vertebrae can go back to their correct positions. The pain signals being created by squeezed nerves, nerves that suggest that the problem is in the toes, the mid back, or even up by the lungs, will cease.

So many people say, "I just bent down to pick up a paper clip, and my back went out!" The problem is not the weight that was lifted, but the quick, thoughtless, assymetrical manner in which the person bent down in the first place.

It is much better to lower the torso towards the ground by bending at the knees, or by very carefully, mindfully, bending equally with both left and right sides, tightening the psoas to lower the torso and then, carefully, gently, symmetrically loosening it again as we stand back up.

To treat a psoas spasm, first make sure the patient's spine is as straight as possible. (See "spinal traction, in the previous chapter, P. 123.) Then, have the patient, who is lying down, bend one knee, with his foot flat on the table.

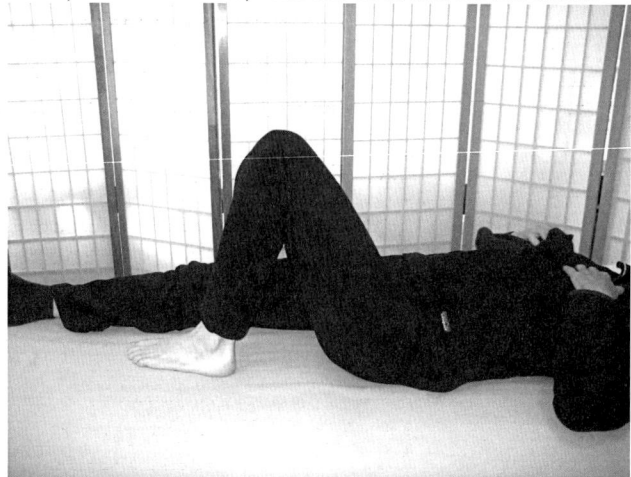

Fig. 13.1 Knee bent, foot flat on the table

The patient or the health practitioner should gently press down with his fingers at the psoas release point: midway between his belly-button and the superior (closer to the head) end of the ASIS (the front part of the hip bone that sticks out in front on slender people.

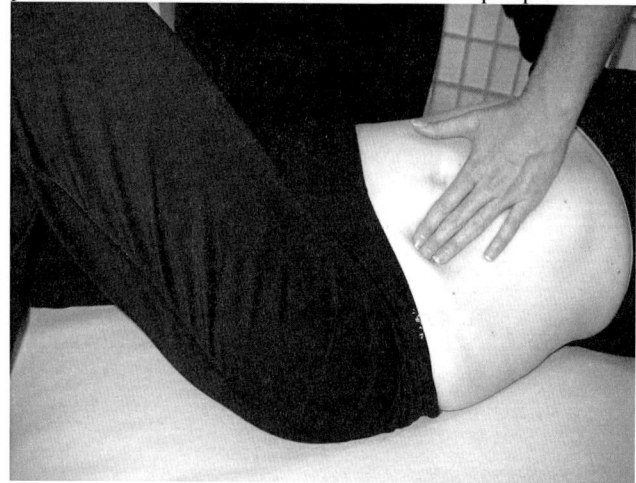

Fig. 13.2 Psoas-release point: mid-way between the belly button and the ASIS

While massaging this psoas release point on his abdomen, he must simultaneously move his bent knee towards the midline of his body. The "midline" is an imaginary line that travels from the nose, down past the belly-button, ending between the feet. This imaginary line divides the body into left side and right side.

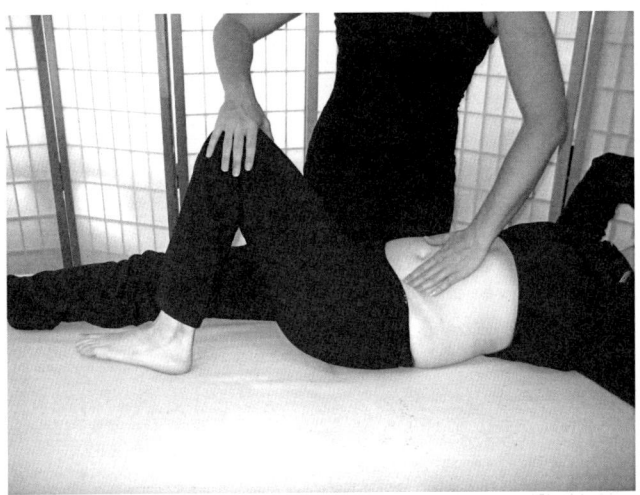

Fig. 13.3 Starting position: knee bent, fingers massaging the psoas-spasm point.

Again: the patient or the practitioner then brings the bent knee gently towards the midline and gently back to its original upright position, all the while massaging the psoas release point on the abdomen.

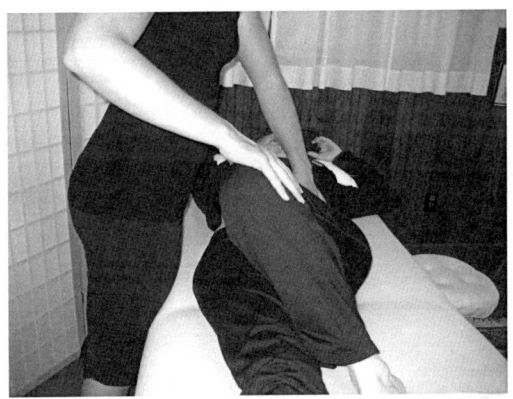 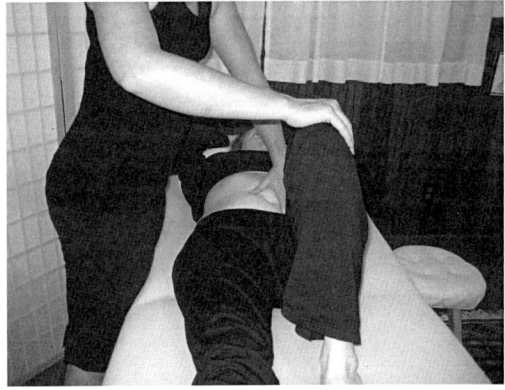

Figs 13.4 and 13.5 Bringing the knee to the midline and then returning it to upright, while massaging the psoas-release point.

Repeat the "knee-to-midline and then back to upright" movement ten times, massaging the psoas-release point the whole time. You should spend about one second on each of the midline-to-upright moves.

After doing this ten times, *then* you may test your treatment by *gently* moving the bent knee out towards the side (laterally). Do *not* force the knee out to the lateral side. It should move laterally more easily than before. If a psoas spasm is very tight, it may still be difficult for the patient to move the bent knee laterally, but it might be easier than before. After doing the above psoas relaxation technique, the patient may suddenly find it far easier to move the knee laterally than it has been in a long, long time. However, if the knee is still unable to move laterally easily, without forcing it, repeat the above.

With a few patient with very tight psoas spasms, I've had to repeat this release sequence for half an hour before the muscles have started to relax.

Psoas release part two: releasing the compensation mechanism

As mentioned in the previous chapter, a person with a psoas spasm will usually have a compensating spasm somewhere else in his body – a compensation designed to enable the eyes to be horizontal with the ground. This compensating spasm is typically in the temporal bones, thought it can sometimes be found in the shoulder, neck, or upper torso.

After the psoas muscle has been relaxed, then you can oh-so-gently rotate the temporal bones to get them to stop being in spasm. After performing the psoas release *and* temporal release on the patient, teach the patient how to do this to himself. He should do both the psoas and temporal releases at least twice a day. Since he needs to lie down to do these, suggest that he do them when he's already lying down: before he gets out of bed in the morning and when he goes to bed at night.

This little "trick" can be enormously helpful. So many people have aches and pains in their back, side, head, neck, or while taking a deep breath, and so on, pains that are being caused by a psoas muscle spasm.

If the spasms quickly resumes after the patient stands up from the treatment table, then you have one of two situations going on: either the compensating spasm was not located in the temporal bones, and you will need to track it down by holding, with FSR, the shoulders, neck, and upper torso. Or, the vertebrae are out of alignment, forcing the psoas back into spasm. If this seems to be the case, and it may well be, with severe spasms, you may want to redo the psoas sequence a few times and then traction the spine a few times, as taught in the previous chapter. After tractioning, perform the psoas release again a few times.

This little exercise is one of the most important tools in my acupuncturist's tool box. I find myself teaching this exercise to patients several times a week. If they are dutiful about practicing it twice a day, their back problems will quickly resolve and not return, even if they have a long history of their backs "going out."

Chapter fourteen

When and where to perform Yin Tui Na

While much of this chapter applies to treating people with Parkinson's, it is also directed at a larger audience: acupuncturists or other medical professionals who are wondering when Yin Tui Na might be appropriate for patients *other* than their PD patients.

As noted earlier, Yin Tui Na techniques are *not* limited to the unhealed foot/ankle injury that is typically seen in people with Parkinson's disease. They can be used to treat any physical injury, whether recent or old, in any patient. The exception is an injury in which some body part has been extremely dislocated and therefore needs strong, physical pressure (*Yang* Tui Na) to be restored to its correct location. For example, a dislocated shoulder (ball of the humerus) needs to be physically moved back into position. But less overtly displaced injuries may respond well to more Yin techniques of Tui Na.

The three most common questions that arise at the acupuncture college where I teach are 1) *when* is Yin Tui Na indicated, as opposed to treating the patient with therapies such as acupuncture, herbs, laser, magnets, sound, and so on, 2) *where* is Yin Tui Na indicated, particularly in cases where pain at a certain location might be triggered by an unhealed injury at a *different* location. How can I determine the location of the root cause – and is that the place to perform Yin Tui Na, or should I treat the painful area and ignore the root cause? And 3) *how much* time, or how many treatments will be required to solve the problem?

When to perform Yin Tui Na on a patient

If a patient has pain that seems to be related to an *injury*, some Yin type of Tui Na is often a good first step in treatment/diagnosis.

The simple act of using one's hands on the injured area, with supportive pressure, will reveal whether or not the body part in question is *able* to respond in the normal manner.

If the patient's injured area yields a normal, reflexive response to supportive touch, Yin Tui Na is probably not *needed,* even though it might be pleasant and might accelerate the healing. But so long as there is normal responsiveness in the injured area, that area has the capability of self-healing. In these cases, other therapies, such as acupuncture, physical therapy, light, sound, herbal therapies, a simple, cheap, ace bandage, or even just the passage of time might be all that is needed, depending on the injury.

However, if the patient's body does *not* perform a normal, reflexive response to supportive touch, it is very likely that acupuncture, physical therapy, and so on will *not* be particularly effective in dealing with this particular injury or trauma - yet.

If the patient's injury area has tissues that are broken or twisted and/or the micro-muscle in the area is holding tight to prevent further injury, acupuncture or herbs will not necessarily reset the broken bone or unwind the twisted fascia. The micromuscle tension that is holding the injured mess in place will not necessarily loosen its grip in response to being attacked with acupuncture needles, cups, or lasers. However, the holding pattern *will* usually loosen up in response to human support that temporarily takes on the job of stabilizing and protecting the injured area.

When the patient's injured area is being protected and held immobile via the hands of the Tui Na practitioner, the patient's body can relax its protective grip. The patient's body can then assess the injury or trauma, and begin healing it.

Only when the post-injury tension in an injured area is relaxed are any displaced or twisted body parts able to drift back to their correct positions. But when the area *has* relaxed, and the damaged bits have realigned themselves, these body parts can then commence any healing and reconstruction that needs to occur.

In almost any clinical situation where the patient has physical pain from injury, some application of Yin Tui Na is appropriate. It might be FSR, or craniosacral work, or fascia unwinding techniques. Whether the pain is in a "tight neck" or sciatic nerve compression, there is nearly always some structural problem underlying the rigidity or pain. By "structural problem," I mean that some tissue, muscle, or bone has become somewhat displaced or is being held rigid by micromuscle. In most cases, acupuncture and/or herbs, alone, will not restore the displaced or tensed tissues to their correct and relaxed positions. Of course, once the structure is restored, then acupuncture, cupping, and/or herbs may be of great help. In most cases involving structural damage or displacements, the patient will heal much faster if some type of Yin Tui Na is used, initially.

For example, back pain responds to acupuncture. However, many visits are usually required to see full healing or even significant improvement. If the underlying structural displacements and micromuscle tensions are resolved first, and then the acupuncture is added to solidify the treatment, patients typically recover, or are significantly improved, in a mere one or two treatments, on average (based on my limited experience).[1]

As an aside, it is impossible to generalize as to "how much" Yin Tui Na might be needed for treating the infinitude of possible back pain problems. In some cases, starting a treatment session with twenty minutes of Yin Tui Na, and ending with acupuncture, might be appropriate. In other cases, one or two sessions of nothing but craniosacral work, with possibly some psoas release work, might be best. In long-term, severe cases, several sessions of nothing but simple, "boring" support might be needed to bring the body into some degree of correct structure, after which several sessions might be needed in which a few minutes are spent on some type of Yin Tui Na, with the rest of the time being used for acupuncture. If there is significant tissue damage, herbal treatment might be helpful, as well – once the basic structure has been restored.

In general, if there is any possibility of structural displacement, including bones, soft tissue, or even mental holding of micromuscle protection, treatment should begin with some type of Yin Tui Na.

---

[1] Studies abound regarding the efficacy of acupuncture in the treatment of back pain. In many of these studies, it appears that six treatments is considered about *average* for the resolution of back pain. To my mind, six is far too many treatments for an average. In my limited experience, the use of Yin Tui Na (usually some variant of a craniosacral protocol), prior to the acupuncture, can *greatly* reduce the healing time, even for *severe* back pain.

132

If, after structural irregularities have been treated, the channel Qi fails to revert back to its correct, parasympathetic flow patterns, then acupuncture might be used to restore correct channel Qi flow.

If the structure is restored and the channel Qi is once again flowing correctly, the body will be able to quickly heal itself. If significant amount of tissue damage occurred, herbs may be helpful in getting rid of the debris and swelling (referred to as Breaking up Blood Stagnation) and, later on, providing tonics for growing new tissues.[1]

The house building analogy

When building a house, the framing goes up first. Then the wiring. No one ever installs the wiring *before* the framing.

Structural repairs in the body are like working on the framing. These repairs require physical, hands-on techniques – Tui Na.

Electrical repairs – fixing channel Qi aberrations – can be done using acupuncture and even herbs.

Sometimes, if there is no physical impediment such as scar tissue, the "electrical repair," the restoration of correct channel Qi flow, will resume automatically, following the structural repairs. In these cases, the Tui Na alone will have been sufficient to bring about both the structural repair and the electrical work.

Fix the framing before fixing the wiring.

Broken bone example

If someone comes to you with a compound fracture, with his broken bone sticking out of his skin, you don't start treatment by inserting acupuncture needles in his arm. To do so would be like fixing a wiring problem without first fixing the framing.

It is obvious that, when someone presents with a compound fracture, you set the broken bones, first. Then, *after* the structure, or "framing" has been fixed up, or at least restored to correct position, *then* you work on restoring the disrupted energetic support to the area: you can then restore the correct flow of channel Qi by using acupuncture – if necessary. In many cases, restoration of the correct positions of the structure allows the channel Qi to automatically resume its correct flow. Often, no needling is necessary.

In the compound fracture example, the order for the sequence is obvious: fix the structural problem, then restore the energy flow to the area. The principle remains the same even when the structural component is far more subtle: frozen shoulder, a kink in the neck, ear ringing, foot pain. In all of these cases, the healing will occur far faster – if at all – if the structural component is treated first. After the structural problem is resolved, the energy flow

---

[1] As a reminder to any acupuncture students reading this, remember that tonics should *never* be used so long as the injury is still in place. Breaks or displacement of the body's structural components constitute an "Excess" condition. We never use tonifying herbs or perform an acupuncture treatment that will bring more channel Qi into an area where there's already an excess (including blocked Qi, Blood Stagnation or rebellious channel Qi). However, as soon as the underlying displacements ("stagnation") have been resolved and correct channel Qi flow patterns have been restored, *then* tonification with herbs or needles might be helpful, especially in cases of extreme injury or constitutional weakness.

in the area can be corrected or amplified, if necessary, with acupuncture or with visualization on the part of the patient.

Then again, because many patients go to see an acupuncturist expecting to get needles, it can be courteous to insert a few needles, whether or not the underlying structure has been completely restored, or the patient is still dissociated from the injury. In such a case, choose to needle channels that are not affected by the obstruction, so that you will not make the error of "tonifying an excess (injury) condition." Points such as Yin Tang, usually far removed from the point of injury, are usually harmless. However, to use *only* needles in a situation that would be far better treated with a combination of Tui Na and acupuncture is dereliction of duty.[1]

---

[1] I know acupuncturists who confidentially brag that they never "put their hands on" a patient. I know others who warn their colleagues, "Never do any hands-on work or body work of any kind. If you do any body work at all, the patient will enjoy it so much that they'll *always* want you to do it!" Some practitioners have a snobbish attitude against using their hands: they consider that acupuncture is more sophisticated; Tui Na is a "lower class" type of treatment. Others have financial reasons for disdaining hands-on therapies: you can only treat one patient at a time if you're doing Tui Na; you can treat six patients an hour if you never do anything but needles and you let your interns do the moxa. Sad to say, I even know *teachers* of acupuncture and Asian medicine who propound these needle-only beliefs and attitudes.

Happily, in my own few decades in the field I have seen an increase in the number of practitioners who understand that the patient's needs come first. These practitioners, who provide the slow, time-consuming Tui Na when necessary, also generate an extremely high degree of customer loyalty. In my own practice, I've had patients who've temporarily used other practitioners at the acupuncture college, when I've been out of town. They come back to me as soon as possible, with remarks such as, "He never even *felt* my neck to assess the painful place," or "She didn't pay any attention to *where it hurt!* She just stuck needles in!"

Puzzled acupuncture students often wonder why their theoretical studies don't lead to treatments that really do the job. Very often it's because the treatments they observe, and perform, in a college of Asian medicine, are designed to develop their *acupuncture* skills and their familiarity with the classic "illness patterns" related to herbal medicine. By learning this material, they are most likely to pass the licensing exam, a noble goal. *But* acupuncture and/or herbs may not actually be the best treatment for the patient's very specific needs.

Very often, injured or traumatized patients will benefit more from Tui Na, prior to or instead of acupuncture. Without Tui Na, the patient may *not* heal as quickly. Certainly, the Shen disturbance (mental/emotional trauma) part of a serious injury can best be addressed by first using Yin Tui Na to gently bring the patient's attention to the traumatized region. Failure to do this leads to slower healing – if any. However, this form of therapy is utterly ignored in many training clinics. The primary focus in many schools of Asian medicine is acupuncture. This is understandable: the primary focus of the schools *must* be training their students to pass the acupuncture board exams. A Tui Na practical is *not* included on the board exams.

Very often, at colleges of Asian medicine, most of the faculty is highly trained in acupuncture, and not particularly comfortable with performing Tui Na. Sadly, many schools have *one* teacher to teach the required Tui Na class, and *one* teacher for the required massage class. Meanwhile, the *clinic* instructors are acupuncturists who often have little or no interest or proficiency in body-work. So even if the students take a few classes in bodywork, but rarely have a chance to observe it in clinic, or practice it on their patients under the clinical teacher's protective eye.

The above is not intended to put acupuncture schools in a bad light – it is to serve as a warning that a licensed acupuncturist may not be very experienced in Tui Na unless he has gone out of his way to make it a specialty.

Summarizing *when* to use Yin Tui Na

If you are a lay reader, planning to help friends or family members by performing Yin Tui Na techniques to help support an injury, you don't have to worry about what other options might be best. However, if you are a health practitioner, you must be able to decide what kind of treatment(s) will be best for each individual.

In California, an acupuncturist might be trained to carry many tools in his kit: herbs, acupuncture, Tui Na, dietary counseling, or energetics (Tai Qi, Qi Gong, visualization, etc.). What is not taught, enough, is deciding which of these tools to use.

Of course, we learn in school that the age and constitution of the patient, as well as the nature of the problem, will help determine what type of therapy is used.

For example, young children and infants are nearly always treated with gentle, skin-rolling Tui Na, and almost never given strong acupuncture needling. Very old people also benefit tremendously from the human touch of Tui Na, prior to any needling. When working with pregnant woman, you should use Yin Tui Na and needle "mild" acupoints. If stimulation at one of the stronger, "Qi-shocking" acupoints, such as LI-4, is called for, use very gentle acupressure, instead of needling.

Even so, some students graduate with the idea that, in general, acupuncture should always be tried first, and the other options should be used if the patient doesn't respond after many, many acupuncture treatments. They have forgotten one of the first rules of Chinese medicine (dear lay reader, please forgive me while I slip into Chinese medicine slang): "Never tonify an excess condition."

An injury, being (more slang) Blood Stagnation, is *always* an excess condition. In nearly every case, inserting a needle into some acupuncture channel will increase – tonify – the flow of Qi in that channel. If the Qi is running backwards, the needle insertion will increase the power of the backwards flow. If your patient feels a ferocious electrical jolt and breaks into a cold sweat, it is highly likely that you have needled into a channel that was severely blocked or running backwards…and you have just made his situation worse.

If you want to avoid violating one of the most basic precepts of Chinese medicine, the rule to "Never tonify an excess condition," Yin Tui Na is very often the first modality of choice *any* time that tissues, including muscles, bones, tendons or ligaments, or even organs, are displaced.

Yin Tui Na can also be used for other types of problems with an *injury origin*, such as headaches, vision and/or hearing problems, sinus problems, stiffness, digestive problems, and numbness, to name a few. In all these examples, the underlying root cause might be injury, spasm, or structural displacement – excess conditions, all.

(Warning: here comes more Chinese medicine slang.) Oppositely, if the above problems are being caused by pathogens (Evil-Wind), Excess Cold, Heat, or Damp, or any of the other, non-injury root causes, an approach other than Yin Tui Na might be better. The health practitioner *must* diagnose the root of the illness in order to know which treatment modality to use.

Yin Tui Na can be helpful if a patient is trying to consciously rid himself of emotional (Shen disturbance) problems brought about by any of the seven "Pernicious Emotions (fear, anger, melancholy, anxiety, excess sadness (self-pity), worry, hysteria, and fright (panic)." The hands-on support of various forms of Yin Tui Na, together with the focused effort of the patient, can be extremely effective.

People with emotional traumas buried in their past very often hold tension in their neck, lungs, diaphragm, liver or heart area, to name just a few holding spots. By applying hands-on support to these and other soft tissue areas, a therapist using Yin-type Tui Na methods can often initiate healing of problems such as asthma, insomnia, indigestion, or other maladies and pains, if these problems were stemming from traumas being retained in the soft tissue – so long as the patient is also working on changing the mind-set that allowed the tension to be retained.

Yin Tui Na is probably *the* most effective clinical means of treating a disorder in which the patient has mentally *dissociated* from the trauma. If the patient has dissociated, no number of needles, no number of herbs, will break through the mental barrier formed by the patient.

Old, unhealed injuries very often occurred in life-threatening situations, or situations in which a person would put himself at risk if he ever revealed his injury.

For example, a person who breaks his leg while fleeing from a crazed knife-wielder may be able to run for miles on his broken leg. If, after attaining safety, he maintains a dissociated mindset from the terrifying event, the leg may not heal – nor will he ever feel the pain of the broken leg. He may develop knee and hip pain, or other health problems because of the long-unhealed condition. However, these pains may appear to be utterly unrelated to any long-forgotten, unhealed leg injury.[1]

An important diagnostic tool

A very simple way to determine whether or not the patient has constructed a mental barrier is this: ask the patient to imagine light and energy in some healthy part of his body (the tip of the nose is *usually* a safe spot, unless there is a history of injury to the head). Next,

---

[1] I have come across many doctors and health practitioners who do not believe that any person can have an injury and not feel the pain of it. However, neurologists have long recognized that certain injuries, inherently life-threatening, do *not* manifest pain, at first. Spinal cord injuries, removal of a limb, and stroke are three types of injury that do *not* hurt for the first few days, and usually, for much longer than that.

In the case of spinal cord injuries, approximately 75% of patients begin to feel the delayed pain between 72 hours and one *year*. The remaining 25% might feel the pain sometime between one year and several decades following the injury – or never. Years after a spinal cord injury, long after all movement function has been restored, a person may suddenly experience the classic pain of spinal cord injury: terrible pressure in the head, ripping pains in the neck and shoulders, searing pain in the hips or legs (depending on where the spinal cord was injured) – and may have no way of knowing that this is pain that was experienced during the injury and put "on hold" in the brain until such time as the person had the leisure and safety to deal with it. In the case of stroke, the pressure in the brain actually causes pain, but this pain is "put on hold" in the brain and does not register, in many cases. However, some people do experience the pain of pressure in the head many months or years after having a stroke.

The pain at the severance site of a removed limb may not occur for several weeks or several years after the removal of a limb. (This is different from the phantom limb experience in which people register sensations from the missing limb.)

In my own acupuncture practice, unhealed, long-forgotten injuries are very common, and are often at the root of a movement disorder.

136

ask the patient to imagine the same amount of light and energy in the injured area. If the patient finds that the injured area is dimmer or less able to be illuminated and energized, the patient has created a mental problem: some degree of dissociation from the injured area.

Where to perform Yin Tui Na on a patient

How do you locate the place on the patient's body where you will begin your application of Yin Tui Na?

Of course, if a patient complains of ankle pain after recently turning his ankle, you will put your hands on the ankle area. If he's recently broken his radius, you'll hold his arm at the point of fracture. These are the easy ones.

But patients often insist that there has been no injury at all, or no injury in the problem area. Sometimes, the patient has just forgotten the injury. Other times, the patient dissociated from the injury, and cannot remember it. Sometimes, the pertinent injury is not mentioned because the root injury was in a different part of the body from the current pain, and the patient doesn't see any connection – hence no reason to mention the significant injury.

Very often, the place that hurts is *not* the same place as the injury that lurks at the root of the problem. For example, sciatic pain in the ankle or leg may arise from tension in the hip area (putting pressure on the sciatic nerve) in order to hold the body fairly rigid...so as to protect a forgotten or now painless *neck* injury.

Oppositely, ear ringing *usually* has its origin halfway down the body...in a psoas muscle spasm in the lower half of the spine that is triggering a compensating twist in the temporal (over the ear) bone.

As another example, frequent sprains in the ankle along the Gall Bladder channel may have their origin in a *head* injury along the Gall Bladder channel, a head injury that's causing deficiency (weakness) along the length of the channel, but only showing up in the weak ankle. Then again, frequent sprains might have their origin on the Stomach channel.

And dystonia in the arm and shoulder on one side of the body can be set in motion by protections of an injury from the *opposite*-side arm and shoulder.

Another example is the manner in which problems in the vicinity of Ren-1 or Ren-2 may be the result of injury, long ago, at *Du*-26. After all, the Du and Ren channels mingle during their internal passage down the gastro-intestinal tract, and a glitch in one of these two channels can cause a corresponding glitch in the other one, which manifests when the channels emerge from the anus and begin, once again, their flow towards the head.

Given that just about any injury, if unhealed, might trigger compensations nearly anywhere in the body, how can one possibly hope to know where the keystone injury, the basic, underlying, root cause, is located?

As an aside, I realize that some of the above may seem obscure, or off-topic, for the person who simply wants to learn Yin Tui Na in order to treat the feet of a friend with Parkinson's disease. But by including these few extra examples this book can be a more complete text for acupuncture students, whose patients might present with an infinite array of problems.

Where to begin treatment

Very often, the patient's pain or problems are not in the same location as the unhealed injury. Many people with Parkinson's have neck stiffness or hip pain, but the root cause is an unhealed foot or ankle injury. Until you treat the root cause, the other pains and problems will not go away for good.

Treat everywhere

Some methods of Yin Tui Na address this unknown-location problem by treating as broad an area as possible, on the assumption that, by treating everything, you're bound to hit the problem area, as well.[1]

For example, most schools of craniosacral therapy teach a multi-step protocol in which every bone in the cranium, spine, and pelvic girdle, plus a few of the ribs and the clavicles, are supportively held, however briefly. This approach is moderately *thorough*, but also causes much time to be somewhat wasted – time that might have been better used by directing one's attention to the exact, specific location. Then again, by touching a large range of locations, the main point of injury and the subsequent compensation areas are all addressed during one session. If you aren't able to discern the root location, the site of the original unhealed injury, it's reasonable to take the sweeping view and touch on as many areas as possible during the first or second session with a patient.

Many practitioners who've done craniosacral therapy for many years eventually realize that, in any given patient, they only need to focus on a few of the holding positions – the areas that have no response or only a vey weak response. But they learn this only after some hands-on experience – or else by learning, right from the beginning, how to recognize when responses from a specific body part feel "right" or feel "wrong."

If you know where the exact location of the injury is

Even if you know where an exact "point of injury" is, that place might not be the *only* location that needs treating.

Continuing to use the example of craniosacral therapy, sometimes a patient knows exactly where the injury occurred, but it's no good to just treat that location. For example, a

---

[1] For students of Asian medicine, be aware that pulse diagnosis will probably not help you know *where* the root of the problem, the unhealed injury, is located. For that matter, as most students of Asian medicine quickly learn, despite the assurances of their theory classes, a person with pain from physical injury (a form of Blood Stagnation) does *not* necessarily have a wiry pulse, just as a person with a wiry pulse does *not* necessarily have pain from Blood Stagnation. For that matter, a person who has dissociated from his injury is likely to have a very deep, almost unfindable pulse – the very opposite of the "wiry pulse" that theoretically accompanies injury or pain.

As for tongue diagnosis, Blood Stagnation from injury is only rarely reflected on the tongue. Many people with what you'd call "Blood Stagnation from unhealed injury" have perfectly normal tongues and tongue coats, or their tongues reflect some other condition unrelated to the unhealed injury.

person who falls backwards on his head may know perfectly well that his injury occurred to his occipital bone. However, the force of the blow may have caused displacements or twisting in his other cranial articulations, his cranial fascia, his neck, and even his lower spine. The force of the blow to the occipital bone will probably have traveled to the front of the face, particularly the sphenoid bone, and may have traveled into the neck, particularly the upper cervical vertebrae. From there, the force of the blow may have also become distributed to the frontal bone, the temporal bones, down the spine to the lumbar vertebrae, and into the sacro-iliac joint.

In a case like this, the practitioner will want to give support, and the opportunity of restoration, to all of the affected bones and soft tissue. In this case, even though the injury was highly localized, performing an entire craniosacral protocol, touching on all of the areas with repercussions from the injury, will best meet the case.

Which still leaves the question open: how do we know where to start applying Yin Tui Na, if we don't know exactly where the pain or problem is coming from?

Use Tui Na to find areas that don't respond

Using Yin Tui Na diagnostically was discussed in an earlier chapter: by learning how a healthy body part responds to supportive touch, and learning to recognize the unresponsiveness or incorrect responses of an unhealed, injured area, a Yin Tui Na practitioner can hold the patient's body in many locations, testing for responsiveness. By spending a few moments in many locations, he can quickly zero in on the area or areas at the root of the problem – even if the root is at the opposite end of the body from the patient's pain.

Even if the area with an abnormal response is only a "branch" of the problem, and not the root area, treatment of the branch very often leads the practitioners hands to move, intuitively, quickly, to the root. Performing Yin Tui Na and "listening" to the signals coming from your intuition can be an excellent way of knowing where Yin Tui Na is needed.

Feel the flow of channel Qi, looking for aberrations

Another skill is feeling for errors in the flow of channel Qi. The location of a glitch in the flow of channel Qi suggests an underlying problem at that location – even if there is no obvious pain coming from that area. Knowing how to feel channel Qi, directly, by hand, can be of enormous benefit when looking for an unknown root cause. Once a person has mastered the easy-to-learn art of feeling the actual channel Qi flow, he can assess the patient's entire body in under five minutes. (See: *Tracking the Dragon* footnote, page 61.)

Learn the most common compensating mechanisms

Another skill set that can help in determining the location of the root problem is memorizing the most *common* compensating mechanisms. These most common compensations account for a majority of the problems seen in clinic. A short collection of very common situations in which pain is perceived in one part of the body but has origins elsewhere was already listed earlier in this chapter. That list included sciatic pain, ear ringing, dystonias, and frequent ankle weakness.

How long before the injured body part responds to FSR treatment?

How many treatment sessions will be required?

This technique can work very quickly, within minutes, for a very recent (in the last twenty-four hours) injury, in which the patient is no longer in danger.

Oppositely, with injuries that have been ignored for decades, and particularly if the patient, at the time of injury, *decided* to deny the pain and injury (dissociation), the injury might not release for weeks, months, or years (assuming one-hour treatments once a week).

I had a Parkinson's patient whose feet needed three years of intermittent FSR therapy, with approximately fifteen to twenty treatments a year, before he was able, suddenly, to move his ankle, wiggle his toes, feel his feet, and all other normal foot functions.

On the opposite side of the time-frame spectrum, a person with a recently (in the last 48 hours) broken bone may respond to FSR within minutes – even if the bone has already been set, and is already encased in hard plaster. Which brings up the subject of broken bones. Yin Tui Na was often translated as "Bone Medicine," in the past.

Broken bones: an aside

If a broken bone is already encased in a cast

Even if a broken bone is already encased, application of FSR, with supportive hands resting on the *outside* of the plaster or plastic cast, can allow the twisted tissues inside the cast to relax and "reset" themselves, perfectly. If the injury was very recent, the injury can often be restored to health within minutes. It is very rewarding. It can also be perceived as "miraculous" by the patient, who can usually feel the bones moving around "spontaneously" inside the cast.

In these cases, it becomes clear that the electromagnetic support from your hands is doing as much, or more, than the actual physical contact of your hands.

This technique can help the broken ends of the bone realign themselves *perfectly*. This perfect alignment is similar to the way in which broken porcelain can be set back together so exactly that the seam is invisible, and a faint electrostatic bond between the porcelain pieces tentatively holds the pieces into place.

When this perfect reset can be brought about in a broken bone, through the use of FSR, the broken bone often stops hurting, the tissues around the bone stop hurting, and healing can be extremely rapid.

I've known patients (patients who did *not* dissociate from the pain) to be able to walk on a broken foot or ankle bone in three days, with no casting, by having received FSR treatment within several hours of the injury.

Toes and collar-bones

Typically, a western doctor will not bother to reset a broken toe. Even with a broken collar-bone (clavicle), the doctor often just puts the arm in a sling and doesn't reset the collar-bone itself, unless the bone parts are significantly displaced. These injuries are usually left to "heal themselves." They rarely heal correctly. The toe or collar-bone may be torqued, and a source of pain, for the rest of the patient's life. If you can treat such an injury within a few days of the injury, before the break has begun to knit with an incorrect alignment, you can use Yin Tui Na to help the bone ends restore themselves to their exact correct position, and save the patient from a lifetime of nagging pain.

When bones "refuse" to knit

Also, in cases of a bone that has been casted but has failed to knit, even after one or two periods of the typical six-week wait, application of FSR can support the injured area so that the area relaxes enough to eliminate the twisting in the soft tissues that was keeping the bone ends apart, and releases the static forces in the tissue that remain as a result of the injury. As soon as these forces are resolved, the ends of the bones revert to their original positions, bringing the broken edges close together in a perfect fit. Once this occurs, knitting of the broken ends commences immediately, even in bones that had been failing to knit.

If the patient is wearing a cast, place your hands on the cast and leave them there. Soon enough, the patient will feel "something going on" in the vicinity of the break.

Of course, if the emergency room or orthopedic MD has made things trickier for you by putting a few "pins" in the bone to hold it in place – without first having released the tension in the surrounding soft tissue – it may be nearly impossible to help the bones reset themselves. The tension in the soft tissue, together with the tension that the physician introduced to the tangle, *all held in place by the pins*, will usually prevent the bone from knitting quickly and easily, and no amount of Yin Tui Na will be able to get rid of those pins. If you can get the surgeon to remove the pins, you will have a much better chance at helping the patient heal completely.

Chapter Fifteen

A definition and history of Tui Na

This chapter might seem a bit extraneous, even redundant. It might well have been placed near the front of the book, as additional introduction material. However, I placed this non-crucial information here at the back to allow readers to more quickly cut to the chase and get started on actually practicing Tui Na.

The following information won't teach you perform Tui Na, but it might help you feel more knowledgeable and comfortable about the subject of Tui Na in general.

What is Tui Na?

If the hands of the practitioner make contact with the patient' skin or the patient's clothing, the practitioner is doing Tui Na.

When a doctor repositions a patient's dislocated shoulder, the doctor is doing Tui Na. When a chiropractor adjusts spinal bones, he is doing Tui Na. When a craniosacral therapist gently cradles the skull while feeling for the movement that pumps cerebrospinal fluids, he is doing Tui Na. When a shiatsu practitioner stimulates acupoints with his fingers, sometimes referred to as acupressure, he is doing Tui Na.

On the other hand, techniques such as Reiki, in which the hands hover over the patient but do *not* make contact, are *not* Tui Na. Energetic distance healing is not Tui Na. Techniques like acupuncture, moxibustion, or cupping, in which needles, moxa, or cups make contact, but the hands do not play a major contact role, are *not* Tui Na. Acu*pressure*, however, which is digital stimulation of acupressure points, *is* a form of Tui Na.

Bodywork styles range from powerful to subtle

Hands-on bodywork can range from the strong-arm tactics used to replace a dislocated shoulder to the simple, firm, supportive holding of a panicked newborn baby.

All forms of body work can be placed somewhere on the spectrum that ranges from "very vigorous, directed, and visible to the naked eye" to "very unobtrusive and/or undirected." "Undirected," in this case, means no directional intention on the part of the practitioner.

For example, Rolfing, Swedish massage, and the "bone-crunching" style of *some* styles of chiropractic work, are at the vigorous end of the spectrum. Oppositely, "Craniosacral therapy," "Therapeutic Touch," "Unwinding," "Zero Balancing," "Bowen therapy," and the many other trademarked "light touch" therapies that are proliferating today are near the unobtrusive and/or undirected end of the spectrum.

In Chinese medicine, the terms "Yang Tui Na" and "Yin Tui Na" are used to define the two ends of the hands-on therapy spectrum. Yang Tui Na refers to those techniques at the vigorous, visible-to-the-naked-eye end of the spectrum. Yin Tui Na refers to those techniques at the light-touch, unobtrusive or undirected end of the spectrum.

More about Yin techniques

Some Yin techniques can be so subtle that very often an outside observer might think that nothing is happening: no one seems to be moving or being moved. Some light-touch, Yin types of Tui Na are almost imperceptible to the patient. Some use no overtly directed force, but work on the principle that mere manual support of an injured person or injured body part can help stabilize an upset area or bring about the relaxation that allows innate restoration of displaced tissues back to their healthy positions. "Mere" manual support may even trigger the initiation or acceleration of healing by helping a person shift away from sympathetic mode (fight or flight mode) and back into parasympathetic mode ("relaxed mode," a mode in which healing is able to occur).

Between Yin and Yang

Some techniques are in the middle of the spectrum, not particularly Yang nor particularly Yin. For example, pediatric skin rolling, in which the skin of an infant's back is gently pulled away from the torso, in a rolling motion that travels from the skin near the neck down to the skin near the hips (or from the hips to the neck), is *mildly* active, inasmuch as the patient's skin is being actively moved. However, there are no particular bones, muscles, or tissues being targeted. This technique is neither extremely Yang nor extremely Yin, but is somewhere on the middle of the Tui Na spectrum – it might be called "mildly Yang Tui Na."

Acu*pressure* is another example of a hands-on technique that is not particularly Yang and not particularly Yin.[1] Acupressure consists of gentle rubbing or pressing at the spot where some acupoint is located, in an attempt to stimulate channel Qi to move forward through an area that has insufficient flow of channel Qi. Like pediatric massage, it could be referred to as "somewhat-Yang" Tui Na. Then again, if the acupressure is somewhat subtle, it might be better described as "somewhat-Yin" Tui Na.

The psoas release technique presented in this book is mildly Yang inasmuch as it is an overt, visible directed movement – but even so, it is very Yin in comparison to most other psoas release techniques.

All forms of hands-on body work, whether they were first written up in China, Sweden, or Beverly Hills, can be placed somewhere on the spectrum between Yang Tui Na and Yin Tui Na. In other words, Tui Na is not a term that refers to a specific technique for adjusting the neck or calming a frightened child. Tui Na is an umbrella term. It refers to any type of *hands-on* bodywork.

Legal notes

Acupuncturists in some states are required to take one or two classes in Tui Na to complete their degree in Asian or Chinese medicine. In many schools, the Tui Na classes

---

[1] "Acupressure" is a form of Tui Na, and has nothing to do with needles.

The word "acupressure" is a misnomer. "*Acu*" is from the Latin, and means "needle." The word "acupuncture" means "*puncture* with a needle." The word "acupressure" literally means "*pressure* from a needle." Which it is not: it is pressure from a hand, or finger. It should be called manupressure, or something like that.

Presumably, someone who had no idea that the prefix "acu" means needle came up with the word acupressure to describe pushing with fingers. The word acupressure has come into common use, however. Nothing to be done about it now, I suppose.

144

teach only very Yang Tui Na techniques for specific bone displacements, injuries, pains, or weaknesses.

However, certifying laws in many states allow a licensed acupuncturist to perform Tui Na, without stating what *types* of Tui Na he can perform. This means that a licensed acupuncturist, in such a situation, may have only studied Yang Tui Na moves in school, but he can legally perform craniosacral therapy: a light touch, Yin Tui Na type of bodywork, and bill it as a form of Asian manual therapy. By definition, since craniosacral therapy uses the hands, it is a type of Tui Na.[1]

Historical note: the disappearance of Yin Tui Na

More than twenty years ago, as I was studying for my Master's degree in Chinese medicine, I came across a book in the school's library titled *Tui Na: Chinese Massage*. This book was purported to be a direct translation of the text approved for use in one of the top Chinese Medical schools. (The poor quality of the translation – a characteristic of all the recently translated texts, at that time – made a convincing case for this claim.) The book started by stating that Tui Na is an ancient art, preceding the development of acupuncture: "The unearthed oracle inscriptions ...of the Shang dynasty record that the female witch doctor, Bi, could treat patients with massage [Tui Na]."[2]

The introduction of the book then proudly explained that both Yin and Yang forms of Tui Na were a part of the rich cultural heritage of China. It explained further that Yang techniques were overt, and were usually used when an injury was new and painful ("bright," or "Yang"). Yin techniques were subtle. They were more likely to be used if an injury was old, forgotten, and painless ("old," "dark," and "hidden" are all "Yin" qualities).

The introduction went on and on for several pages with generalities about the difference between Yin and Yang, together with repeated assurances that all known techniques, ranging from Yin to Yang, would be presented in the book.

However, when I flipped through the book, I discovered that the introduction was incorrect. The book contained only *very* Yang techniques: overt twisting of the spine to

---

[1] The gross generality of referring, for acupuncture licensing purposes, to all hands-on bodywork as "Tui Na" leads to much confusion. Many people looking for a health professional to perform Yin Tui Na on an injury have discovered that some health practitioners touting "Tui Na" in their yellow pages ads very often have no idea that *Yin* type techniques even exist. When these practitioners studied "Tui Na," what they actually learned was an assortment of techniques best described as a sampling of *Yang* Tui Na.

For another example of confusion that arises by thinking that "Tui Na" refers to a specific type of bodywork, in Texas, sometime around year 2000, a judge suggested that Tui Na be removed from the scope of practice for acupuncturists. He was upset after seeing two cases, in one year, in which poorly trained acupuncturists had performed neck-cracking (chiropractic type) Yang Tui Na... and broke their patients' necks. The judge, not understanding that "Tui Na" means, essentially, "any hands-on therapeutic touch," wanted to make Tui Na illegal. Technically, this would have outlawed all forms of touch on the part of acupuncturists, including feeling pulses (an action which, by mere contact, *can* slightly alter a patient's condition). I have no idea what the current law is, in Texas.

[2] *Chinese Massage*. Publishing House of Shanghai College of Traditional Chinese Medicine. Shanghai. 1988. p.2. Note: the Shang dynasty dates from approximately 1766 BC to 1027 BC. The actual text would have said that Bi could treat patients with *Tui Na*. Again, the use of the word "massage" when translating into the English is not accurate.

relieve back pain, violent snapping motions of the neck for displaced cervical vertebrae, and so on.

There was no mention anywhere in the book about gentler techniques such as skin-rolling, acupressure, or the deeply supportive, gentle type of holding that can bring together and reset, perfectly, painlessly, the ends of a broken bone, or the firm support that can bring the patient's attention, and therefore healing, to an injury that had been long ignored.

I pored through that book, looking for any Yin techniques. I inquired in the school's office as to whether the Yin techniques might be in a separate volume. No, there was no missing volume. This was a translation of the entire book, the official version of government approved medical Tui Na.

I learned, a few years later, that *Yin* Tui Na had been dropped from the Officially Approved Texts although it had been left, most likely by accident, in the *introduction* to the texts. This disappearance probably occurred because, at some point in the twentieth century, the light touch therapies were deemed "not scientific enough," and even "too charismatic" (related more to the practitioner's charm than any medical science). At any rate, by government decree, Yin Tui Na was no longer taught. Officially, it no longer existed.

My own medical practice just happened to develop in a direction that required the application of *very*-Yin Tui Na. I was working with patients with Parkinson's disease, many of whom had dissociated from terrible injuries.

As mentioned earlier, these patients had injuries that had never hurt – or had "never occurred" – usually because of an ongoing traumatic situation in which the injury was the lesser of two troubles.

Very often, patients did not want these injuries touched by me, or by anyone. Many patients, terrified at the idea of therapy in the injured area, informed me that "No one has ever touched my left foot." Or, "I never even let my spouse *look* at that part of me."

In order for me to gently draw the patient's attention to these wounded areas, thus ending decades of dissociation, I found myself using extremely Yin Tui Na: nothing but very firm, utter support wherein I placed my hands on either side of the injured area and simply held it for an hour at a stretch, once a week, until the displaced tissues began to move of their own accord under my hands, or until the patient suddenly exclaimed something like "Ouch! My ankle feels smashed!"

Although, years earlier, my shiatsu professor had referred to this type of holding simply as "support," without providing an Asian name for his technique, I was thrilled to read, in the introduction of *Tui Na: Chinese Massage,* that Yin Tui Na was the Traditional Chinese Medicine name for the "support" work I had been doing on "old, painless, forgotten injuries" in Parkinson's patients.

Based on the hiatus in the book, it seemed that the techniques I instinctively used to treat these injuries, derived from the "support technique" I'd learned in the Shiatsu class, no longer had an official place in the *modern* Chinese medicine cannon. Certainly, these techniques were no longer being taught in the Chinese schools of Tui Na.

The teacher of the "support" techniques I had learned in school had stressed *supporting* with the hands, as opposed to manipulating with the hands.

In 1998, when I first wrote up an article about the results I was getting in treating people's "painless" injuries, my article briefly described the hands-on technique I was using.

The editor of the journal was brilliant, detail-obsessed, and gloriously nit-picking. The *American Journal of Acupuncture* is now defunct, but at that time, it was the most respected, longest-running English language journal of Chinese Medicine. The editor told me that the hands-on technique I was describing was a "Yin" type of Tui Na.

I'd had no idea. After all, the only book I'd ever seen that even mentioned the words "Yin Tui Na" in the intro had included *no* information about Yin techniques in the text.

Still, the book had said that Yin Tui Na was used when injuries were old, painless, and even forgotten. That fit my patients to a tee. I accepted the editors assertion, and from that point on, in my medical practice, I referred to this work, and any light-touch variations such as craniosacral therapy, as Yin Tui Na. Happily, this gave me the convenience of keeping all my hands-on treatment modalities under the vast umbrella of the Chinese medicine term "Tui Na." This also kept all my treatments under the umbrella of the legal "scope of practice" of an acupuncturist: in California, an acupuncturist's scope of practice includes Tui Na.

I was happily surprised to see how my patients responded to this new label for the work that I'd been performing on with them. Before I knew to call the holding technique "Yin Tui Na," I had been merely holding their injuries in some very slow, boring, albeit effective, fashion. But now, when I could casually mention that the technique being used was "a Yin form of Tui Na," they *loved* it. They could even search for "Tui Na" on their computers and get results, so they knew I wasn't just making things up. I no longer underestimate the power of a name.

Nearly ten years after that first article was published in the *American Journal of Acupuncture*, after I'd published books describing Yin Tui Na techniques and had lectured on the subject in the USA and abroad, I was thrilled to learn, from an acupuncturist attending one of my lectures, that people in China were, once again, *openly* using Yin Tui Na techniques. I cannot verify this student's report, but he said that, for many long years, the subtle Yin forms of hands-on healing work had been banned from the official medicine – but health practitioners had continued to perform it in secret. Now, at the beginning of the new millennium, I learned that Yin Tui Na was, once again, being practiced openly as a medical procedure.

By the early twenty-first century, as China basked in the burgeoning international support for acupuncture, Qi Gong, and other esoteric practices that had all been banned in China at one time or another (because they invited mockery from the more "scientific" western countries), even subtle medical techniques such as Yin Tui Na were once again out in the open.

I do not know if Yin Tui Na techniques have regained their rightful place in the Chinese medical schools and text books. I do hope that the written material regarding Yin Tui Na was only locked up, and not destroyed. At any rate, we westerners can now state with assurance and confidence that hands-on healing techniques at the more subtle, less intrusive, less-directed (Yin) end of the spectrum are in fact techniques of Chinese medicine, just as much as the bone-snapping, body-jerking (Yang) forms. For acupuncturists, in many states and countries, these gentle forms of support are allowable according to our scope-of-practice laws: laws that permit us to perform "Tui Na" but which don't specify what types of Tui Na.

More history

Shortly after I graduated, I asked the Chinese doctors and teachers at my California acupuncture college for their definitions of Tui Na. My teachers were all practicing acupuncturists. One teacher, an MD in pediatrics from Shanghai, said, "Tui Na means pediatric finger massage: skin rolling." An MD/ Ph.D. in Chinese medicine from Guan Dong said, "It means all forms of Chinese massage." An MD from elsewhere in southern China said, "It cannot be translated. Tui Na means Tui Na." An MD from Shanghai said, "It means bone medicine." Another MD from Shanghai said, "It means bone massage."

My friend Sue, who was an accountant in southern China and now owns a Chinese restaurant in California, gave this non-medical translation: "Tui Na is a doing word, it is a word that means you do something, and then there is a result. It means moving, doing, and then it brings something out that wasn't there before. So then you have something. Because you did something, this way." She moved her hands in a slow, open and shut, back and forth pattern to demonstrate.

Back in the 1980s, when I started working on a Master's degree in Chinese medicine, the most common classroom definitions of Tui Na were "bone medicine" or "skin rolling/pediatric massage." The latter is a relatively new meaning of Tui Na, going back only to the Yuan dynasty. During the Yuan period (1271-1368), the Tui Na/massage department of medicine came under the administration of the bone-setting department. A department of pediatrics was opened also and incorporated into the Tui Na department, making "skin rolling techniques" an official part of the government-approved Chinese medical protocols.[1]

Today, as mentioned earlier, Tui Na is the name given to almost any form of physical-touch work in which the doctor makes intentional hand contact with the patient. Technically, even acupressure, a process in which acupoints are stimulated by finger pressure, should be considered a form of Tui Na. As for the bone-setting applications of Yin Tui Na, it is almost never used in western countries. In western countries, the re-setting of broken bones is nearly always done in a western medical clinic or a hospital's emergency room.

The proliferating field of light touch therapies

This section has been included because so many correspondents have written to me that they feel nervous or even inadequate with regard to performing Yin Tui Na. No matter how many times I write, "This is simple holding; a child can do it," I get frequent emails saying, "What if I'm doing it wrong?" or other phrases suggesting failure to master the subtleties of this tricky business.

I want to reassure every reader that, even if a light touch technique has a name, like "FSR", that doesn't mean it is necessarily technical, magical, or needs to be studied under the auspices of some authority. And in the case of FSR, it's almost impossible to do it "wrong" unless you aren't holding firmly enough.

---

[1] *Chinese Massage*. Publishing House of Shanghai College of Traditional Chinese Medicine. Shanghai. 1988. p.12.

To help understand this, consider that many of the modern, light-touch techniques that can be placed under the broad umbrella of Yin Tui Na have their own, special names, even though many of them are based on very, very similar principles. In the vast panoply of light-touch therapies, it is sometimes impossible to say where one named technique leaves off and another begins. In the last thirty years, it seems as if dozens, maybe hundreds, of therapists have been busy developing new "unique" versions of light-touch therapy and slapping their own names or a copyrighted trademark onto some variation of human touch. Some of these techniques claim to be unique because the hands are allowed to rotate a bit, compared to techniques in which the hands move in a linear fashion. Other techniques claim to be unique because the emphasis is on very short periods of touching or mere brushing against the skin, as opposed to touch that lasts for longer periods. However, for all these techniques, the underlying principles are universals, and not "inventions."

As an interesting legal point, techniques cannot be copyrighted. *Names* for techniques and the specific *text* used to describe them can be copyrighted, but, actually, the act of touching a person in a therapeutic manner cannot be copyrighted or patented.

For example (becoming a bit far-fetched, but helping to make the point), holding a person's hand can be considered a form of hands-on healing. There are many ways to hold someone's hand. An inventive person could, if he wanted, make up a specific name for the variation of hand holding that involves, say, interlocking the fingers. He could name this finger interlocking after himself and copyright that *name*. This would *not* mean that this person discovered or invented the interlocked finger position. By law, he could *not* copyright the *technique:* he could *not* demand a royalty payment from anyone who linked fingers. Nor could he prevent anyone else from writing about the technique of linking fingers – so long as that other person used his own words and a different name, if any, for the technique. Which is to say, so long as the other person does not plagiarize.

He could, however, publish books on the subject and hope that people would, from then on, choose to refer to themselves, whenever they interlocked their fingers, as doing the popular "Wilson Hold," or, depending on his name, of course, it might possibly be the "MacGruder Support" or the "Spongeworth-Hugeusson" Technique (if two people wrote it up). This might provide a temporary sort of name recognition and fame, and possibly some book sales. But just the same, the actual performance of interlocking fingers, also known as "holding hands," cannot be copyrighted.

I suspect that most of the exciting and new techniques that are flooding the field of light-touch therapy are, despite their copyrighted names, nothing more than the normal, intuitive touching and responding that emotionally healthy humans can do automatically – behaviors that are becoming more acceptable as our culture moves away from the rigid, "don't touch yourself or others" mores of the past.

I am certain that if we modern humans, yes, even doctors, spent more time practicing touching in an intuitive, healing manner, the way that most of us rub, pat, and hold our pets, we would realize there is nothing new about the miraculous "new" light-touch healing techniques that are so hot right now.

Not only that, I suspect that we *all* know how to do these techniques, already. Reaching out to one in pain is an innate function in most of the mammals. Weirdly, we humans are usually *taught* to not touch ourselves or others, according to cultural constructs.

But if we can overcome these "rules" that have been imposed on us, we find that we already know how to hold and encourage healing in others with our hands.

Oddly enough, since we tend to *touch* very little and *feel*, or I might say *perceive*, even less, some members of the modern generations of would-be health practitioners choose to take extra classes to learn *basic, core* medicine: how to touch, how to feel, and how to support with our hands. But most health practitioners, including MDs *and* acupuncturists, even after several years of medical school, have never learned how to touch and hold a patients' injured or insulted body parts in a supportive, constructive manner.

Sadly, even after years of training, many health practitioners, both eastern and western, do not even know how to recognize which of a patient's maladies might best be treated by some type of hands-on therapy.

Fortunately, many of the researchers who are experimenting in this field are doing a brilliant job of writing about those techniques that work for them and publishing case studies. Of course, writing about this realm of light-touch therapy can be challenging: it can be as difficult to describe in words just what a touch technique should feel like as it is to describe in words the flavor of an orange.

Despite this difficulty, a few of the people who are writing about these new techniques are working hard to make their writing available for free or at low cost. Some have done an excellent job of promoting light-touch work, offering frequent workshops and promotional material to "get the word out." Others have worked hard to explain, using terms from biology, physics, metaphysics or by making up new words, just how these therapies work.

And many patients who have *not* responded to conventional western (allopathic) medicine have benefited from some of the new light-touch therapies.[1]

In English, we do not have a widely accepted medical umbrella term that covers all the schools of light-touch therapy. Therefore, they are each considered to stand alone – some even consider themselves as competing with one another. By referring to all the light-touch therapies as Yin Tui Na, by putting all of them under the same over-arching banner, it's easier to describe how the various light-touch techniques differ, and how they are similar. The differences, of course, can be as infinite as the human imagination and vocabulary allows. The similarity is that all these techniques employ the hands of the health practitioner in a supportive manner, in a fairly unobtrusive and/or somewhat undirected manner, in direct contact with the patient's skin.

---

[1] A study undertaken in the mid 1990s revealed, much to the astonishment of the allopathic medical world, that one third of the people in the US had used "non-traditional" medicine. The alarming thing was that a majority of these people had never told their doctors for fear that their doctors would respond with anger. Of all the "alternative" modalities, acupuncture is the one most requested from people seeking alternative medicine coverage from their health insurance companies. Strangely, hands-on therapies, including massage, are also very popular, but are almost never considered to be "medical." Unless the hands-on therapy is being done by a licensed Physical Therapist, it is usually dismissed as "feel good" treatment, and is not covered by insurance or deemed "significant" in resolving a biological problem.

But most important, and the purpose of the above rant, is to assure you that *you* can do this work.

That's it.

Whether a person is doing nothing but simple holding, or doing some of the "fancy" hand position holds of craniosacral therapy or the relatively quick, reflex-stimulating movements of Bowen work, the basic precept is *touch*, with, usually, some amount of supportive holding and, sometimes, fairly subtle movement, suggestions of movement, or even imagining movement. And that constitutes "Tui Na."

Many of these simple techniques are innate. We see mothers with their babies doing these exact same techniques, automatically, to keep their babies comfortable and happy. When the infant is upset, the mother holds the baby snugly. When the infant is hurt, the mother kisses the spot and holds it, and at some point, starts to gently test the injured area. Sometimes, the mother gives just the lightest hug or jostle, at some tense spot, and the child's tension melts.

However, in our culture, we are taught, at an early age, never to touch others except in specific, culturally approved ways. For many of us our innate understanding of how to hold the traumatized areas on another person's body has been squelched. [1]

In learning the various forms of Yin Tui Na, and especially FSR, all we are really doing is relearning something that we already know: how to give support with our hands in such a way that an injured or traumatized person can most quickly resume responsiveness and self-healing.

It's that simple. It's also extremely powerful.

---

[1] When I was attending high school in a highly urban area, I met a new student with whom everyone quickly felt very comfortable. If a classmate was stressed, the "new boy" would unself-consciously lay a comforting arm on a shoulder, or give just the right amount of pressure in a reassuring hand-hold. I was amazed at how he seemed to generate ease and comfort among whomever he socialized with. I asked him where he was from. He was from a small rural area in Michigan. His family had kept dairy cows. Since his earliest days, he'd spent his mornings and evenings among the cows. After I got to know his family, I realized that all of them had the same, slow, gentle, comforting way. He had never been trained in "light touch" therapy. He did it instinctively: he touched people the same way that he'd touched cows.

Chapter sixteen

How I learned Forceless, Spontaneous Release

Shinzo Fujimaki

When I was getting my master's degree in Traditional Chinese medicine, classes in Tui Na/massage were required. I was fortunate to have classes with one of the most brilliant "massage" therapists in, I think, the world. I put the word massage in quotes because the class that Shinzo Fujimaki Sensei was teaching was officially titled "Shiatsu Massage." However, what he taught us was nothing like the usual acupressure poking and prodding that is normally associated with Shiatsu.

Master Fujimaki was so famous for his "massage" therapy that his appointment calendar was always booked at least three months in advance. His clients testified that his treatments had removed problems ranging from chronic pain to cancerous tumors, asthma, and a long list of other "incurable" ailments.

As a teacher, he worked very hard to convey to us the essence of what he was doing. Many of my fellow students did *not* like his class. Their complaint usually ran something like: "He is wasting our time telling us about his ideas. I don't get it. I just want to learn where to push to cure which problems. Fujimaki never tells us anything we can *use*."

But many other students, myself included, considered our classes with Master Fujimaki to be some of the most important foundation-stone hours of our entire school career.

Shinzo Fujimaki was a man with a radiant smile. He was also an aikido master. When I saw him, now and then, striding along the cliff tops of our ocean-side city, his walk evoked images of tigers and horses. To best honor what he taught, I will quote to you, as closely as I remember, the words he told us, over and over. It will be up to you, as it was left up to us, to see if you can find anything helpful in his words.

Support, support, support

"Support, support, support.

"If a patient is lying on the table, and you push down hard on them giving acupressure or massage, or push hard when you are feeling for the right place to put the hand or the needle, his body will automatically push back against you. There will be a fight going on. How can a person relax, how can he begin to heal, when he is fighting? If the patient is lying on his stomach, do not push his back down into the table. Instead, put one of your hands under his chest and your other hand on top of his back. Position the upper hand directly over your hand that is underneath. Now when you push on his back with your upper hand, resist that push with the hand that is underneath. That way, you are doing all the work; you are doing the pushing *and* the resisting. Your bottom hand is supporting the patient, holding him strong against your push.

Support, support, support. You give the support; then the patient doesn't have to work at resisting you or work at supporting the weight of your hand. The patient can be peaceful, he doesn't need to resist you; you are resisting yourself with your opposite hand.

"The patient cannot relax if you are pushing or poking him. If your goal is to allow the patient to relax so that he can let go of his problem, do not hurt him. Give him support. Support, support, support.

"If you are going to have one hand on [some body part of the patient], your other hand should be on the other side [of the body part], catching the power of your first hand, protecting the patient from your active hand. If you are not doing any pushing, if you are just resting your hand on a patient, still, his body will have to worry what to do about your hand. His body will be pushing back on your hand, especially if you are touching a part of his body that is scared.

"But if you support the patient by putting your other hand on the opposite side of his body [part] to support the patient, and use that other hand to catch the energy from the first hand, then the patient can relax. Sometimes both hands are active. Sometimes both hands are supporting. It doesn't matter. The only thing is this: the patient should not have to do *extra* work because you are imposing on him. The patient should be allowed to relax. Support, support, support."

Have fun

The master continued: "My attitude when I am giving treatment is that I am having fun. I learned that I gave the best treatments after I had already worked about eight hours. After working eight hours without a break, I start to feel hungry, tired. I cannot stay focused on my work even if I try. I begin to think that I cannot survive if I don't stop working. My mind becomes distracted from my work. I want so much to stop working that I cannot think about what I am doing. To keep myself going, I imagine that I am looking up at the blue sky. I imagine that I am at the beach.

"I love to go to the beach. When I go to the beach, I imagine that I am a red horse, a red pony, and I run in and out of the waves. When I am finished running in and out of the waves, I lay on the sand and look up into the blue sky.

"When I am starting to get so tired from treating clients, after about eight hours, but I can't stop because there are still more clients with appointments for several more hours, here is what I do: I think that I am lying on the beach, looking at the sky. I have discovered that during this time, when I am exhausted and looking at the sky, when the sky exists and the patient is no longer the center of my focus, *this* is when I begin to give good treatments. After a few more hours of still working hard giving treatments, when I am *in* the sky, when I *am* the sky, when the patient doesn't even exist anymore, then I am starting to do the best treatments. I learned this.

"So now, whenever I *start* working, I put my mind on the idea that I have already been working eight hours. I think that I can no longer keep going. I must start to imagine that I am looking into the blue sky. My idea is that I am so completely drained, I am so tired, I cannot think anymore about the patient. I can only survive if I am, in my mind, looking up at the sky with all my love and energy."

Shinzo-san often worked twelve and thirteen hour days without taking a break. His point, however, was *not* that he gave his best treatments at the end of a long day. His point was that he had learned that, no matter whether he was just starting his day or was starting on his twelfth client, his mind must always be as desperately seeking transcendent joy as a drowning man seeks for air. When he could hold his mind in this state, the treatments – no matter when they were scheduled – more or less took care of themselves. Meanwhile, what were his hands actually doing? Support, support, support.

154

Every week in shiatsu class, when he demonstrated his techniques on volunteer patients, I watched his hands. Where was he placing them? Very often he would start with the hands on the part of the patient's body that was having pain. But just as often, as he gently pushed, vigorously pushed, or let his hand rest on the patient's skin - always with his other hand giving oppositional support – his hands would gravitate, with almost no conscious thought or motive, to some other part of the patient's body that seemed to want to be held, pushed, or prodded. When he stopped thinking about what his hands were doing, his hands knew automatically just what to do.

Even if one of his hands then pushed or prodded, the patient never responded as if he was being pushed or prodded. The patient usually didn't seem to feel much of anything, except safety and relaxation, because the actual work of Shinzo-san's hands was somewhat undetectable to the patient's reflexive tendency to push back. Why? The support, support, support that his hands were giving each other.

Some of my fellow students resented this general talk about support, support, support. They kept asking him highly specific questions like, "Where's the best place to push on the patient for asthma?" or "What point should I use for acid indigestion?" They missed the point that the patient's own body would show you where the important blockages were. They resented the idea that the "curing point" for asthma or for indigestion might be in different locations on different people. They wanted simple, one-size-fits-all location-formulas to cure the various Chinese medicine diagnoses of their patients.

I only mention this because, if you are looking for someone to do Yin Tui Na, you cannot assume that an acupuncturist, or even someone who is certified in Asian body work, will necessarily be knowledgeable about or even interested in the slow, hands-doing-the-diagnostics style of Yin Tui Na.

Control your thoughts

Another point that Master Fujimaki made was also very important, although I fear many of my fellow students only thought that he was relating a funny story.

"In Japan, we have a massage tradition that the patient leaves his clothes on. When I first came to this country, I was surprised that people remove their clothes for massage therapy. I was not used to working on bare skin.

"After I had been working in this country for about a month, I felt very bad about the way that my American patients behaved towards me. After every treatment that I gave, *every* treatment, the patient told me that he wanted to have sex with me. I thought that this was very bad. Young men, young women, old men, old women, they were all the same. After the massage, they all wanted to talk about having sex with me. I thought this was an American habit.

"One day I decided to learn why this was happening to me. I realized that I had a cultural difference about bare skin. To me, because of my Japanese background, bare skin suggested having sex. I must have been conveying my cultural ideas to the patients. So I made an effort to understand that in this country, bare skin was not a statement about having sex. I never again used this wrong idea about bare skin during massage.

Ever since that day, when I changed my attitude towards bare skin, not once after a treatment has finished has a patient wanted to talk about having sex with me, not *once*.

"When my mind was on sex, every patient thought about sex. Now I think about the red pony and the blue sky, and my patients think about whatever they want; and they recover from their pain and the sadness that was holding on to the pain."

I could write volumes about this shiatsu class that taught us "nothing" about classic shiatsu. However, I think the above examples make the two points most important to our work with Parkinson's patients. First, the patient must be supported. No matter how much or how little energy the health practitioner is applying to the patient's body, the patient should not feel the need to fight back or resist any of it. The patient should not need to push back unless he, for some reason, wants to. The support, support, support that Shinzo-san insisted on creates a pressure-free, supportive environment for the patient's body, as if the therapy, no matter how vigorous or how firm, somehow seems forceless *to the patient*.

The other important point is that the mental sojournings of the practitioner are important. The best results occur when the practitioner is not trying to give undue influence to the patient. If the practitioner's mind is focused on something, the patient can pick up on it and even misinterpret it. Even focusing on healing the patient is usually inappropriate: if the practitioner is focusing on healing the patient and the patient is holding back for some reason, an unspoken conflict ensues. In the throes of this conflict, the patient cannot let himself go, he cannot relax. The patient cannot attend to the business of healing if he is busy fighting the practitioner or defending himself, however silently and invisibly.[1]

But when the practitioner forgets about trying to heal the patient and plunges himself headlong into his own joy or inner peacefulness, the patient is less threatened. The patient can let his guard down. When this happens, the patient's body may very well start doing what it was designed to do: heal itself.

My 1989 class was the last year to have Shinzo Fujimaki as a teacher. The school administration, after receiving several complaints that: "Shinzo doesn't teach us anything *real*," replaced him with a teacher who told the students, right out of the texts, just where to push on various acupoints and how hard.[2]

---

[1] When I wrote this sentence just now, I realized that it sums up, very well, the problem that Parkinson's patients are dealing with. *A person cannot relax and cannot let go if he is busy defending himself, however silently and invisibly.* Keep this phrase in mind as you work on your PD patients: do not judge him, do not try to mentally "help" him or pray for him. Mentally, *leave him alone.*

Of course, you can always pray for him after the session is over and you are not technically working on him.

[2] Of course, this material was redundant; as second- or third-year acupuncture students, we already *knew* all the point locations and their applications. The replacement Shiatsu teacher simply demonstrated that these points could be stimulated by hand as well as via needles, and spent the whole semester doing it. I suspect that a few students liked this format because they didn't have to learn anything new. They could spend the class practicing acupressure on acupoint locations that they'd already studied.

Now that I am teaching at an acupuncture college, I see that *most* of the students are highly idealistic, and want to do what is best for the patient. But I am including these "negative" bits to help the reader understand that, just as all MDs are not the same, all acupuncturists are not the same.

156

Dr. Paul Lee

Fulfilling another course assignment, I was privileged to take a class in Medical Qi Gong from a Qi Gong Master.

Dr. Paul Lee (Lee Pu Long), recently arrived from China, taught a brilliant class in which he taught us very specific techniques that patients could perform on themselves to stimulate their own healing energy in various body parts.

By way of introduction to Dr. Paul Lee, I will describe one of his projects. His work in China on self-applied eye massage had been adopted by the national government and was being taught to Chinese school children. The government had wanted a solution to the problem of poor vision becoming rampant among children at the seventh and eighth grade level. As students were doing increasing levels of book-work, they were starting to need glasses. This is considered perfectly normal in the west, but in China, where the government is the supplier of eye exams and eyeglasses, this trend towards "student's myopia" was considered a problem.

Dr. Paul Lee had devised a quick and easy program of Qi Gong (energy control) that included gentle eye socket massage and using the energized palms of the hands, held a short distance away from the face, to push and pull energy into and out of the eyes. Starting in sixth grade, students did these quick exercises every day at school. They subsequently did not develop myopia and did not need glasses, even as they progressed through the later school years.

This type of Qi Gong exercise, in which the patient learns how to focus on a body part and move energy through it in a soothing, healing manner, is the essence of Medical Qi Gong.[1]

---

[1] Regrettably, some students have embraced a version of "medical Qi Gong" in which the doctor uses his own energetic power to force healing onto a patient. While this may sound appealing to people who like the idea of having power over others, this type of work does not improve a patient's health in the long run. A person who allows his body to be manipulated in this manner actually suffers a weakening of his own will power and sense of energetic direction.

When the treated malady returns (and it will, sooner or later), the patient will be even less able to activate his innate healing energy than he was before. His body will passively wait for the next blast of healing energy from the healer rather than doing its own work. This type of healing, in which a charismatic person refers to himself as a Healer and forces the energy in a patient's body to move in an unnatural (not according the patient's will) manner, is considered very bad form by many traditional Qi Gong practitioners. This type of work can be dangerous to the ego of the practitioner and does no long-term good to the patient.

Great souls from time immemorial have done miraculous healing work. However, these souls performed their healings by removing first the causal (ideational) problem that set in motion the unhealthy energetics: the unhealthy energetics that manifest as the illness. Therefore, these great souls actually do remove the entire illness. More importantly, they only perform these miraculous healings when their cosmos-attuned intuition tells them to do so. They have no personal desire as to whether the person heals or not at a specific time. For the most part, if they have a preference, they prefer that their patients seek the Truth and Love that will enable them, the patients themselves, to cast out their own demons instead of passively waiting to be healed.

Patanjali, a contemporary of Socrates and one of the greatest Hindu writers on religious philosophy, makes his point in his Yoga Sutras. He explains that a sign of spiritual advancement is the ability to remove illness, including the underlying wrong thinking and past karma that caused the illness. But he also makes the point that a truly advanced soul may have this ability and, because of his

This class taught me crucial lessons in the role that the patient plays in healing himself. If I could summarize the essence of the Qi Gong class, it would be this: the best doctor is one who sees where or what the source of the problem actually is, and then shares helpful information, even including specific exercises, to help the patient to change himself. The good doctor may advise on diet, exercise regimen, movement patterns, or instruct the patient in how to recognize where energy is moving incorrectly and how to correct it.

The point of the treatment is to help the patient learn what he was doing wrong that made him susceptible to the illness, and how to correct it. The burden of recovering and staying recovered is on the patient. The job of the doctor is to non-judgmentally figure out the source of the problems in the patient and suggest to the patient a direction that will reverse the problem. The goal is relieving patient suffering through patient education and empowerment, which may include the patient learning some energetic (Qi Gong) exercises or learning an attitude adjustment. A further outcome is the confidence and positive attitude the patient develops as he learns how he can confront his own weaknesses and change them.

Techniques used on PDers

The many classes that I took in Asian and American bodywork, including some of the teaching in the Medical Qi Gong classes, all contributed to my understanding of Tui Na. Some of the techniques I learned in school had names. Some did not. The result of taking these classes, in addition to the other classes required for a Master's degree in traditional Asian medicine, was that I had learned, at least on a beginner's level, how to use my hands in a supportive manner.

When I got my license and started practicing medicine, if I did include Tui Na in the treatment session, I never bothered to mentally define which, if any, particular technique I

---

wisdom, will choose the more difficult path: not using his spiritual powers to force an alteration in a person's chosen life direction unless commanded to do so by God. The truly wise understand the roles that sickness and health play in this worldly drama of cause and effect. The highest role, for a practitioner of medicine, is providing support so that the patient can heal himself.

However, some modern medical Qi Gong practitioners ignore this wisdom from the past. These well-meaning people, finding that they have the ability to temporarily alter a sick person's energy, go ahead and do so, imagining themselves to be spiritual healers. Even worse than the inevitable return of the illness in the original patient, these would-be healers often become deeply sick themselves despite their magic mantras, dramatic hand gestures, and bowls or gimcracks for "catching the bad energy." If this type of Medical Qi Gong healer does get sick, then when his "healed" patient's problem inevitably resumes, there are then two people sick with the same malady. From a larger standpoint, the world is worse off than before. Even if they do not get sick, these would-be healers are perpetrating the false idea that they, and not the patient's own self-directed life force, are the driving component of the healing process.

Only a Self-realized master can truly remove from the cosmos, through exercising his will in accordance with Divine instruction, the wrong energetics in another person's body, mind, and heart. However, each one of us has the right and the ability (usually undeveloped) to instantly or gradually heal ourselves from the results of our own wrong thinking, the wrong thinking that is our own source of our emotional, mental, and physical health problems. In the new testament of the Bible, Jesus celebrated a teaching moment when he pointed out, insistently, that he was not responsible for the healing of the woman who clutched at his robe and was instantly healed. He emphasized that she, and not he, had worked the miracle. The miracle came about through her faith, through the change in her thinking as she willingly tapped into the Love that Jesus personified. Jesus was trying to make the point that all of us have within ourselves the capacity for "miraculous" self-healing.

158

was using on a given patient at any given moment of hands-on therapy. Everything I was doing was the sum of all the things I had learned. I imagine that this becomes true for all bodyworkers: at some point, one ceases to perform "techniques" and just "does whatever needs to be done."

When I started working with Parkinson's patients, I automatically sensed that I needed to use very Yin techniques of Tui Na to both assess their physiology and to treat it. Very possibly my own latent and utterly unsuspected Parkinson's symptoms, including my lifelong aversion to being "messed with," helped guide me in this direction.

Putting FSR into writing

I've already mentioned, in chapter fifteen, that I only found out I was doing Yin Tui Na when I wrote my first article on Parkinson's and submitted it to the *American Journal of Acupuncture*. The editor told me that there was a generalized name for what I was doing: Yin Tui Na.

She also pointed out that Yin Tui Na was a generic term, and for the article, she wanted to use a more specific name for the exact type of Yin Tui Na that I was using.

Then the editor paraphrased what I'd said by saying that the Tui Na I was using was a very light-touch, spontaneous-release type of Tui Na with no intention-based directional movement, which the patient *perceived* as supportive, as opposed to intention-based and forceful. I concurred. So she had me refer to the Tui Na I was using as a forceless, spontaneous-release style of Yin Tui Na, or FSR. She had me include in the article a few details about the techniques to make it very clear that the work was forceless so far as the patient's perception was concerned; it was not directed at any particular response from the patient. If, how, and when the patient responded, it would be some sort of spontaneous healing event on the part of the patient, not a change in response to anything *actively directed* by the practitioner.

The intent of the editor was not to create a trademarked technique. Nor was there an intention of implying that I had ever learned a specific, rarified technique of this name, passed secretly from master to master, through the ages. The editor and I were merely looking for a way to describe, as clearly as possible, exactly what it was I was doing. What I was doing was a Yin type of Tui Na, one that was perceived as pretty much forceless and intention-free, and which resulted in patients having some sort of release whenever they were ready to do it.

Again, I did not invent this technique. I learned everything I know from my teachers. They did not always have a name for everything they taught. My editor, rightly, wanted something more than "holding," and came up with the adjectives "forceless" and "spontaneous release."

After publication, I was surprised by requests from people with Parkinson's looking for referrals for "FSR practitioners," as if FSR was some sort of "official" technique. At that time, I still considered it "simple holding," and only used the name FSR when writing about our Parkinson's research, in order to emphasize that the holding had to be perceived as forceless, non-intentioned, and that the releases, if any, would come spontaneously from the patient and not be "induced" by the practitioner.

By the time I web-published the fifth edition of *Recovery from Parkinson's* in 2000, even I was referring to the light-touch techniques I used on people with Parkinson's as the acronym "FSR." Today, in 2012, when I say "Forceless, Spontaneous Release" or "FSR," my mind's eye now sees capital letters and an acronym where there used to just be plain old adjectives. Somehow, this technique has turned into yet another named therapy!

But keep in mind, this is not a mysterious therapy from the misty past or the distant shores of Asia, but a basic method of using hands to work with an injured person. FSR is not a specific, exacting technique. FSR is just a way of providing support, support, support. Do not worry about doing it "correctly." Just do it, and enjoy doing it.

A frequently asked question

Is there a Yin Tui Na practitioner in my area? Is there an FSR practitioner in my area?

Again, there is no such thing as a *specific* technique called "Yin Tui Na," per se. "Yin," in this context, simply means, "on the gentle end of the spectrum." Seeking a "Yin Tui Na practitioner" is asking for a person who does *any* type of technique that is relatively gentle hands-on therapy, as compared to strong, vigorous therapy.

It does make sense to ask a practitioner who advertises "Tui Na" whether he has studied Yin-style or Yang-style techniques, or both. If the respondent says that he doesn't know, or if he says that he does "traditional Tui Na," this means that he probably has studied only Yang-type techniques. Most people who study Tui Na are studying the Yang type. As a generality, while practitioners of Yin Tui Na are very aware of the existence of both the Yin and Yang kinds, most practitioners of Yang Tui Na are *not* familiar with the ideas of light-touch work.

People who *have* studied the Yin forms of bodywork have usually done so by studying western types of light-touch work. They would be more likely to refer to their techniques by the specific, western names of the particular modalities that they studied. For example, a western, hands-on, light-touch therapist might say: "I do both Gregson's cranio-tarsal work and Marco's Medical Unwrapping protocol," but he might have no idea that these his light-touch therapies are considered to be forms of Yin Tui Na.[1] Simply from lack of bilingual understanding, most practitioners of light-touch bodywork would probably *not* refer to their work as Tui Na. Many western-trained light-touch therapists have never even heard the term "Tui Na."

So the question arises, "Is there a FSR practitioner in my area?"

Probably not. This is a pretty simple, dull technique. Few people get training in a technique of simple holding – a technique that any person can usually master in an hour or two.

So why do I stick with the fancy term "Tui Na"? Why don't I just refer to these techniques, in general, as "simple holding"? I'm licensed as an acupuncturist. That license allows me to do modalities that fit under the umbrella of traditional Chinese medicine – which, by law, includes Tui Na. I am legally able to perform Tui Na. Officially, I am not licensed to "simply hold."

---

[1] Both of these named techniques are fictional, created for the sake of example.

160

Also, no western terminology is as broad as the term Yin Tui Na. By using this term, I am giving myself the widest possible latitude in terms of techniques that are within the scope of my practice – even techniques that are as simple as providing firm holding with no expectations…techniques that *anyone* can easily learn to do, licensed or not.

Getting back to looking for a "trained FSR practitioner," you probably are not going to find anyone. These techniques, though utterly simple, have only recently been written up, given a name, and discussed in the context of treating Parkinson's disease.

You probably cannot find anyone who is familiar with the name FSR unless he is already familiar with our work with Parkinson's disease.

But the FSR techniques can be easily mastered by almost anyone who is able to sit still for several minutes at a time. You do NOT need to find someone who is "experienced" in this technique. Become that person, yourself. You will find many opportunities to use this therapeutic work – and so long as you have your hands, you've got your tool kit with you.

Blessings

Index of drawings and photos